A Wellness Guide©

NATURES BENEFIT FROM CORAL CALCIUM:

Sorting Facts from Speculation

Stephen Holt MD

www.wellnesspublishing.com

Book Cover Design and Typesetting by Asha Azhar.
Manufactured in the United States.
Library of Congress Cataloging-in-Publication Data.
Holt, Stephen 1950 –

Natures Benefit from Coral Calcium: A Wellness Guide.

ISBN – 0-9714224-4-3

1. Coral 2. Health Benefits 3. Calcium 4. Coral Calcium 5. Minerals 6. Longevity 7. Alternative medicine 8. Fossilized Coral 9. Coral Collection 10. Coral Processing 11. Nutritional Medicine 12. Dietary Supplements 13. Bruce Halstead 14. Robert Barefoot

A Note to the Reader:

The author of this book is not attempting to provide advice on the treatment or prevention of disease. Whilst the health benefits of dietary supplements are reviewed, it is not the intention of the author to provide an alternative to the orthodox physician / patient relationship. Rather, it is the objective of the author to expand the dimensions of orthodox medicine itself by provoking more interest in remedies of natural origin. Food is being incorporated more into medical practices in the 21st Century, where diet and lifestyle will play a predominant role in preventive medicine. This book was not written to endorse the use of specific products or for any treatment purpose. The conclusions in this book represent the authors' opinions of medical, scientific, folkloric and lay writings on the various topics discussed.

The publisher and author accept no responsibility for the use of any agents mentioned in this book. Before any individual self-medicates, he or she is advised to seek the advice of a qualified health care professional. The author does not support unsubstantiated claims of health benefits of foods or dietary supplements. This book must not be interpreted as product labeling.

PREFACE

Coral calcium from Okinawa, Japan has become one of the most popular dietary supplements in the US. Consumer confusion about this dietary supplement prevails and clarification about its source, properties and potential biological effects is required. The development of interest in coral calcium as a food supplement reminds one of other phases in the popularization of some nutraceuticals (dietary supplements) where "hype" may have transcended science. This circumstance tends to threaten any valuable category of dietary supplement. A dietary supplement can become damaged by over promotion and the propagation of misleading information. I am not necessarily describing a circumstance where individuals have given intentionally misleading information on the subject of coral calcium. Some opinions on healthcare matters are zealous whereas others are balanced. The enthusiasm for promoting a dietary supplement sometimes overtakes "hard" facts. This has happened and continues to happen with many classes of dietary supplements, much to the detriment of the nutraceutical industry.

In this short book, my writings have moved towards investigative reporting, as I try to educate myself and others on the science of remedies of natural origin. I do not know all the answers to questions posed on the subject of coral calcium; and I must make it clear that my interest in coral calcium as a supplement was fuelled more than ten years ago from an initial position of almost cynical skepticism. My interest in coral calcium has graduated to the point of belief in this dietary supplement as powerful, poorly understood, promoter of health and well- being. In this book, I explore how and why coral calcium could work to benefit health, but I can only speculate on its potential biopharmaceutical actions. Steeped in folklore, arguments, rhetoric and emerging science, coral calcium is playing an increasing role in America's wide array of putative, health-giving food supplements.

There is no doubt that the interest in coral calcium has swept the nation. From humble beginnings as means of purifying water, coral calcium has been promoted in network marketing, radio shows, books, articles and more recently national TV infomercials. In the dietary supplement industry, one witnesses a repeating phenomena with product promotions, where the use of the supplement is driven more by the charisma and personality of the promoters, than it is by the clinical science behind the product. I stress that we have little in the way of controlled clinical studies on the benefits of coral calcium, but there are thousands of testimonials concerning its benefit. Marine biologists have clarified much about the habitat and composition of live coral and its fossilized remnants that have been called "coral calcium".

This book attempts to sort out science (or facts) from speculation on the subject of coral calcium from Okinawa, Japan. When it comes to coral calcium, many people ask, "Where's the beef?" This metaphor refers to a quest for "clear" facts about the health potential and benefits of coral calcium. The many anecdotal reports of the benefits of coral calcium are screaming to be further explored in scientific studies. However, much uninformed rhetoric about its origins characteristics and biomedical applications must be questioned. I have committed myself over the past three years to examine the origin, quality and biological characteristics of coral calcium in order that people may make informed judgments about its use and potential benefit.

There is a risk, as my publishers keep telling me, of writing books that nobody wants to read. There is more than "a measure of truth" in the statement that "the truth hurts". This reasoning should not apply to our quest for knowledge about the benefits of remedies of natural origin. Without open dialogue and rational arguments, there will be no material advances in "natural medicines".

Let me brighten the horizon of this book by stressing that I believe coral calcium to be a valuable, rediscovered remedy of natural origin with potential to promote health and well being. Coral calcium is a natural, holistic mineral supplement that supplies many elements or micronutrients (minerals) that are absolutely essential for the chemistry of life. In fact, the name "coral calcium" does not do justice this remedy of natural origin. Coral remnants or coral calcium appear to have much more to do with general micro-mineral supply to the body, rather than being merely another source of calcium in our diet.

Please read this book with optimism. It will give you some insight into how difficult it is to sort science or fact from speculations (or rhetoric) when it comes to potentially valuable dietary supplements. The nutraceutical revolution is now part of main stream medicine and a much greater burden of scientific proof has to be placed on scientists involved in developing supplements and also on supplement purveyors. I hope this book will encourage people to select the right kind of coral calcium supplements and trust that it may dispel some of the myths and fallacies that have crept into the biomedical application of one of natures greatest treasures – fossilized or remnant coral from the sea and land mass of the Rukuyuku Islands of Okinawa, Japan.

Stephen Holt MD,
September 2002

SORTING THE FACTS FROM SPECULATION

Depending on your preference for surfing the internet or reading popular literature, you will find descriptions of the dietary supplement, coral calcium as both a panacea "treatment" or a "scam". I believe that coral calcium is neither a medical panacea nor a scam. Coral calcium is a valuable, holistic, mineral, dietary supplement which poses many important issues, ranging from discussions about our current mineral-depleted Western diet to concerns about the ecology and future of coral reefs.

In this book, I avoid discussions or claims about the treatment benefits of coral calcium. These claims have become apparent in many other contexts. Instead, I take a hard look at origin of this dietary supplement with a desire to dispel some of the myths and fallacies that have emerged in the description of this valuable, health-giving natural resource.

THE BIOLOGY AND GEOLOGICAL ASSOCIATION OF SEA CORAL

Living coral polyps have a mouth and tentacles that allow these unique organisms to live by consuming plankton. The living polyp secretes minerals, principally calcium carbonate, to form a hard covering or exoskeleton. When the coral forms its "stony house", other coral polyps grow on the hard foundation. This process creates coral reefs which are the largest structures on earth that are built by any living organism.

The distribution of coral in temperate oceans is quite uneven throughout the world. Much coral lives in underwater zones that are adjacent to aggregations of volcanoes or seismic activity. Underwater volcanic activity or the remnants of this activity produce a mineral rich environment in the sea water in which coral lives. Thus, live coral often filters minerals-rich sea water. The changes of climate under the sea or simple wave action causes natural breaks in coral reefs The reefs often shed a sand-like material. This coral sand is supplemented by the excretions of coral munching reef fish, e.g. parrot fish, which eat hard coral for its content of algae. Coral sand is essentially "dead coral" (fossilized) that covers the ocean floors around the reefs. Coral remnants are swept several miles away from reefs and some form islands or land masses. It is this coral sand that is processed to make the dietary supplement coral calcium. Live coral is not used as the precursor of coral calcium-containing, dietary supplements.

Oceanographic researchers have warned of the peril that threatens the survival of coral reefs (see National Geographic Magazine, vol 195, No1, Jan, 1999). Therefore, the whole issue of the environmental significance of using coral calcium as a food supplement has more than piqued the interests of conservationists. However, it must be stressed that coral calcium has nothing to do with live coral, but there is some residual concern about how underwater deposits of coral sand may be collected.

The living coral reefs of the world form a meeting point for many ocean dwellers. It is a rendez-vous for one quarter of all species of ocean organisms. The "evolutionary epicenter" of coral with the most different species of coral exists in South East Asian seas, but coral material can be found in unlikely places. Fossilized coral deposits are found in the midwest of America where it was deposited millions of years ago (e.g. Bighorn Mountains of Wyoming and Montana). "Dead," coral deposits (fossils) are ubiquitous on our planet.

CORAL CALCIUM AND HEALTH?

It was the mid 1980's when I was introduced to the study of marine nutraceuticals by my mentors at Sun Yat-Sen University of Medical Sciences in Canton (Guangzhou), in the Peoples Republic of China. As a visiting Professor of Medicine at Sun Yat-Sen University, I was paired with my counterpart, Professor Liu (since deceased). Professor Liu was the head of digestive diseases and nutrition at this prestigious Chinese University. In our "private" meetings, Professor Liu would "giggle" and tell me fascinating stories about the Cultural Revolution. He interspersed his stories with his ideas about traditional Chinese medicines, and other remedies of natural origin. His passion was to reveal his "health secrets" from the oceans.

As an allopathic physician with a strong belief in pharmaceuticals (since faded somewhat), I expressed my skepticism to Professor Liu. As a "true-believer" in Eastern medicines, he commented on the ability of nacre powder (oyster shell scrapings) to heal peptic ulcer and expressed his beliefs in "coral grains" (live coral and coral calcium) as a panacea for all ills. Several years passed and my interest in marine nutraceuticals waxed and waned, but I became aware of increasing reports in the scientific literature about the power of this or that health product derived from the sea.

My interest in marine nutraceuticals was piqued by the work of the Harvard University scientist and physician, Dr. Judah Folkman and his colleagues whom started to define antiangiogenic substances in nature, especially those found in cartilage of marine vertebrates (shark cartilage). Antiangiogenesis is the ability of a substance (drug or natural agent) to interfere with new blood vessel growth. The findings of Dr. Folkman and his colleagues focused my interest in research on the far reaching, potential health-benefits of shark cartilage and prompted me to research and co-write one of my first popular books on nutritional medicine, (The Power of Cartilage, Kensington books, NY, NY, 1997). Thereafter, my research into marine nutrients (nutraceuticals) became increasingly intense, and I developed several health-giving supplements of marine origin (e.g. purified fractions of fish oil) with cardiovascular and general health in mind (see Holt S, The Natural Way to Healthy Heart, M. Evans, NY, 1999).

Despite my growing interests in ocean-derived, medical remedies, I could never get very excited in the "story" of coral calcium for health. The overriding factors causing my skepticism were the descriptions of "panacea" benefits as a consequence of its use. When panacea claims for the health benefits of any supplement are made, one becomes "naturally" skeptical. Furthermore, I perceived the notable absence of hard-scientific data on the use of coral calcium as a remedy; and I had a stubborn disbelief that stony coral remnants could have many biological effects - they just seemed so inert! My mind started to change when I met or talked individually to a number of people (more than 500) who had used coral calcium and claimed, in earnest, that they had experienced consistent health benefits.

In the mid 1990's, I had read about the drinking of water treated with "tea-bag-enclosed" coral and its beneficial health effects. The habit of drinking water which had been exposed to coral enclosed in tea bags was promoted initially by Scandinavians. My interest in coral was clinched, when I watched a video-tape interview of Dr. Erik Enby MD, a Swedish physician, who related his long term experiences with coral treatments. My mind remained somewhat "boggled" by lack of explanations of how coral calcium could exert a health benefit. I did not embrace Dr. Enby's theories about coral minerals causing body alkalinity, but I could not disregard his descriptions of consistent benefit with its use in many patients with different diseases. What was this stuff (coral calcium) that kept haunting my thoughts and challenging my skepticism?

In 1997 at the Collegium Humanum Congress on High Technology Medicine in Switzerland, I was "curb-sided" by colleagues after my lecture on marine nutraceuticals and interrogated about coral calcium. Strange as it may seen, I did not even mention coral calcium in my lecture and I was quiet unprepared to answer their questions. It seemed like I was being pushed more and more to gain further knowledge on what many had described as the marine miracle of coral calcium. Still somewhat reluctant to "pick up the gauntlet" with coral calcium, I met even more people (especially over the past two years) who kept applauding the benefits of coral calcium.

My fate was sealed when I was invited to a scientific advisory board meeting of a public healthcare corporation and was introduced to Mr. Robert Barefoot. The introduction was brief, but Mr. Barefoot was anxious to share his reason for being present. It became clear that Mr. Barefoot had worked with calcium supplements, in particular coral calcium, and he explained that his presence at the meeting was largely due to the fact that he had played an instrumental role in advising on the "nutritional cure" of prostate cancer affecting the father of the CEO of the hosting company. The alleged benefits experienced by the person with prostate cancer had been largely attributed to the taking of coral calcium (in a form that was collected above ground). My skepticism still prevailed as I reasoned to myself that many alleged alternative "cancer cures" are just figments of imagination.

My intense education had begun. I looked at literature on the geology, formation and biology of stony coral. I found that the biomedical literature on coral was very scant in scientific terms, but very rich in folklore and anecdotes. There are several accounts of the beneficial use of coral extracts beneficial use in the alternative treatment of several diseases. In 1998, I was introduced subsequently to two of Mr. Barefoot's former partners Mr. Andy Bowers and Mr. Clint DeWitt of Coral Inc, Nevada. Mr. Bowers and Mr. DeWitt presented a powerhouse of knowledge and experience about coral calcium, especially in relation to its collection and processing. In particular, Mr. De Witt has been responsible for pioneering the use of fossilized stony coral and other "natural" mineral supplements as a food supplement in the US for about 15 years.

My professional introductions became even more fruitful when my attention was drawn to the work of the famous marine biomedical expert, Dr. Bruce Halstead MD. In 1992, Dr. Halstead MD had written a fascinating book on the subject on the health benefits of fossilized stony coral entitled "Fossil Stony Coral Minerals and their Nutritional Applications". My dialogue with Dr. Bruce Halstead MD was fascinating. Dr. Halstead has an encyclopedic knowledge of medicines derived from marine life. Furthermore, I found some ancillary information about coral calcium (used in a tea bag) and health in a booklet entitled "Why Calcium?" written by Dr. B. Owen (Health Digest Books, Cannon Beach, Oregon).

With growing enthusiasm about the supplement coral calcium, I formed my own independent opinions, and I collaborated with Mr. R. Barefoot on the identification of further information on coral calcium and introduced him to different sources of coral. Some of this information is to be found in the book entitled "Barefoot on Coral Calcium, An Elixir of Life" (www.wellnesspublishing.com). Mr. Barefoot's book reflects Mr. Barefoot's opinion and not necessarily those of other researchers. Since the initial writing of Mr. Barefoot's book more information and observations have surfaced about marine coral minerals (fossilized stony minerals or coral calcium).

I formulated products associated with the likeness of Mr. R. Barefoot and others at clinical grade, in an attempt to form a holistic mineral supplement. Mr. Barefoot had proclaimed that "all coral (referring to all types of coral calcium) is fantastic." The rest is contemporary history. Following radio and TV appearances by Mr. Barefoot and availability of his book on coral calcium (and Dr. Bruce Halstead's book on stony coral minerals), the interest in coral calcium has swept the nation. That said, I emphasize that I do not subscribe to several prevailing opinions on the best type of coral and, in particular, I am reticent to make any claim of a <u>consistent,</u> therapeutic benefit of coral, even though such benefit may exist. There is no doubt that illegal claims about the curative properties of coral calcium have been made in the media.

THE CONFUSION STARTED

I stress that there are many people with interest in coral calcium and there are even more opinions on its value, or lack thereof. The frenetic interest in coral calcium and anecdotal claims of health benefits, which sometimes defy clear substantiation, prompted me to write this short book. It is not my intention to give a fixed opinion on the biological significance of coral calcium or stony coral minerals, because there are many unknown issues concerning coral calcium. That said, it is time to dispel some of the myths and fallacies about coral calcium or stony coral minerals.

I wish to state clearly in this book that Mr. R. Barefoot was kind to acknowledge my support in helping him to write his book (Barefoot on Coral Calcium: An Elixir of Life, www.wellnesspublishing.com). The section of Mr. Barefoot's book that acknowledged my support in preparing the book (Barefoot on Coral Calcium: An Elixir of Life) stated an inability for Mr. Barefoot and I to reach a consensus opinion on all aspects of coral calcium. However, Mr. R. Barefoot and I share the opinion that coral calcium and all forms of coral minerals constitute a very interesting and valuable category of nutritional supplements (regardless of whether or not they are derived from coral sand collected beneath or above sea level). Let me now dig a bit deeper and further attempt to sort some of the facts about coral calcium from the speculation. One may agree that speculation can be misleading.

WHAT IS CORAL CALCIUM?

At the outset, I wish to indicate that "coral calcium" suffers from its own name. Naming coral minerals as "coral calcium" has resulted in considerable confusion among consumers. It has caused healthcare consumers to focus their thoughts inappropriately on calcium alone when they consider the nutritional value of coral calcium (marine coral minerals or fossilized stony coral minerals). Mr. R. Barefoot may have contributed to this confusion by stressing "The Calcium Factor", a title of one of his earlier books which expresses his opinions on the biological role of calcium in the diet and related issues. The book "The Calcium Factor" focuses upon the work of Dr. Carl Reich MD with whom Mr. Barefoot had shared thoughts and opinions more than twelve years ago. I believe that the promotion of a book written and focused on the element calcium (and claiming it to be the key active component of "coral calcium") has led to consumer confusion. I refer interested parties to two books on coral calcium, one by Mr. R. Barefoot and one by Bruce Halstead MD (both available at www.wellnesspublishing.com).

Coral Calcium or fossilized stony coral minerals are a holistic mixture of minerals in variable amounts. In general, the main elements found in fossilized coral or "coral calcium"are calcium and magnesium. Coral calcium in its fossilized form is best called "marine coral minerals" or perhaps "stony coral minerals". The term "marine coral minerals" refers to the fact that both ocean and land based coral material are examples of fossils which are derived originally from a marine environment. Dr. Halstead MD has objected to the terms "marine coral minerals" or "coral calcium" and he prefers to use the terms "fossilized stony coral minerals". Thus, the whole notion (or semantics) of what a fossil "actually is" has contaminated understanding about coral calcium. Furthermore, there is no evidence that one type of fossilized coral (collected beneath or above sea level) exerts more measurable health benefits than another, despite the rhetoric. Mr. Barefoot has been bold in his claims of health benefits of coral calcium, based on testimonials, whereas Dr. Halstead MD has been quite conservative. These matters are covered in considerable detail in later sections of this book.

CORAL CALCIUM IS DEAD CORAL

Coral calcium is a food supplement (dietary supplement or nutraceutical) that is composed of dead coral. This supplement is derived from remnants of living coral that have fallen from coral reefs, as a result of wave action or other natural processes. Over thousands of years, fossilized coral forms islands or mountains of coral. These deposits of coral can be harvested from land based deposits, deep sea deposits and transitional zones that are tidal. As we start to address the location of coral deposits in Okinawa, even the distinction between marine and some types of land based coral becomes unclear. Harvested coral can be treated by special processing techniques and then used as a mineral supplement in the diet. I reiterate that I believe that all dead coral is a fossil, so coral underwater or above sea level or at tidal interfaces is by definition "fossilized". That said, opinion on this issue differs.

OKINAWAN CORAL CARRIES THE CLAIM OF HEALTH BENEFITS

Fossilized coral is found on many coral islands, but the geographic location of coral calcium with the most reported health benefits comes from Okinawa, Japan. Okinawa is a prefecture (province) in Japan, composed of a chain of coral islands (the Rukuyuku Islands). Folklore, anecdotes and scientific literature describes coral from Okinawa, Japan to be health giving. Dr. Bruce Halstead MD, a marine, biomedical expert and physician, has focused on the benefits of fossilized stony coral (collected above ground), whereas Mr. Barefoot has regarded all coral as health giving. Mr. Barefoot is quoted repeatedly as saying that "all coral is fantastic". Mr. Barefoot has promoted the use of tea bag enclosed coral, fossilized minerals and below-sea collected coral with varying opinion over time. More recently, Mr. Barefoot has developed an affinity for extolling the advantages of below-sea coral, but he has not presented clear evidence that it is superior to other forms of coral, despite his assertions (and those of others).

ABOVE AND BELOW–SEA CORAL CALCIUM AND BOTH BENEFICIAL

Upon careful review, I reiterate that I can find no credible evidence whatsoever that one form of high quality coral (collected above or below-sea level) is superior or inferior to other forms, despite unsubstantiated claims to the contrary. The most important characteristics of coral that determine its suitability for use as a food or dietary supplement involve many factors. These include its contents, mode of processing and a consideration of the collection process used to obtain the coral; with special consideration for techniques that will not damage the environment. When coral is used as a food supplement in human nutrition, the avoidance of contaminants in coral calcium (especially ocean pollutants) is very important, Contaminants seem to be more common in unprocessed "deep" sea-collected (under the water) coral (vide infra). In fact, Dr. Bruce Halstead's biggest concern about coral sand collected beneath sea-level is its <u>potential</u> content of pollutants, such as plutonium. This opinion is debated by many interested parties.

WHY OKINAWAN CORAL?

Why Okinawan coral calcium has been favored over other types of coral may be more related to folklore than science. The associations of coral with the robust health and longevity in the Okinawan population are impossible to link causally in a direct manner. Several scientists (especially the proclaimed "Quackbusters") have argued that health and longevity in Okinawa, Japan can only be linked to coral calcium by coincidence. I believe that coral calcium from other locations may be health giving as a mineral, dietary supplement, but this has not been explored.

Some "researchers" have made the absurd proposal that living microorganisms in coral supplements are responsible for its health benefits. Even more preposterous are suggestions that the "microbes" are living in coral that is eaten as a food supplement and that these "living bacteria" exert a favorable effect on the ecology and function of the human gastrointestinal tract. You will learn that coral calcium is processed by methods of "strict" sterilization, often using heat or ozone to render the coral remnants "free" of bacteria and other microorganisms. Further, some processing techniques may involve heating coral to very high temperatures, to drive off heavy metals which are contaminants in some coral, e.g. lead, mercury and organic chemicals (environmental pollutants).

The lines of reasoning about the health benefits of Okinawan coral go something like this: Okinawans live long in relatively good health. Their environment is mineral rich as a consequence of the presence of coral. Mineral enriched environments have been associated with longevity, e.g. mountain populations in Tibet and Northern Pakistan. Therefore, coral is the reason for this observation of longevity among Okinawans. Whilst plausible at first sight, this "apparent", tautological reasoning has to be questioned, but it could be true!, albeit arguably!

Whilst it is true that Okinawans live longer on average than main-land Japanese inhabitants, their lifestyle and diet differs substantially from other populations. Therefore, factors other than coral calcium may promote health and longevity in Okinawans. Whilst mineral enrichment of several environments have been associated with longevity, excessive amounts of specific metals can cause disease. Whilst other factors must operate in the health and well being of Okinawans, coral calcium (marine coral minerals or fossilized stony coral minerals) remains an interesting candidate as an apparent "environmental" contribution to good health in Okinawa.

OKINAWAN LIFESTYLE

Finding and studying populations with longevity (long life and good health) has fascinated medical scientists and anthropologists. It is believed, by some, that studying people who live long will reveal the secrets of long life. Despite many attempts to find the "fountain of youth", the discovery of this kind of an "elixir of life" has eluded all explorers from time immemorial.

Modern concepts of aging have started to stress the importance of healthy lifestyle as a key antiaging factor (see www.anti-agingmethods.com). The lifestyle of the "relaxed" Okinawans may be very different from the urban Japanese. There are many differences in dietary habits, stress levels, exercise, and social habits that can be distinguished between the island dwellers (e.g. Okinawans) and "urbanites". These lifestyle factors may operate variably to determine longevity or premature death. For these reasons, it may be impossible to define the health-giving role of a single environmental agent, such as coral calcium (marine coral minerals or fossilized stony coral minerals).

HOW STONY CORAL FORMS

There are two basic types of living coral, "soft" and "hard-stony" coral. These organisms belong to the same general category of organisms as jellyfish, hydroids and sea anemones. It is the stony type of coral that forms a hard outer covering of minerals (exoskeleton). The elaboration of this outer skeleton by coral polyps (which are themselves soft) takes many years. This process occurs as a consequence of the living coral polyp extracting food and minerals from sea-water. Thus, the contents of coral contain most minerals present in sea-water, which in turn contains most elements or salts available in the earth's crust (including in some cases, some modern industrial "pollutants"). Unfortunately, the coral and other marine organisms will tend to concentrate pollutants from the environment such as heavy metals (e.g. mercury, lead and cadmium) or organic chemicals e.g. PCB's (polychlorinated organic compounds). That said, coral calcium is available for use in dietary supplements in a form that is free of any significant amounts of such pollutants (www.naturesbenefit.com).

All sea dwellers have an unfortunate tendency to be at the mercy of environmental pollution. The issue of toxic compounds in seafood has become a major public health concern, especially in waters abutting mainland Japan. However, the waters around Okinawa are considered quite clean or "pristine" (in relative terms). One must be aware that severe illness from heavy metal contamination (e.g. mercury poisoning) has been recorded close to industrial zones in several Eastern Asian locations, especially industrial areas in mainland Japan. For these reasons, a discussion of sources and types of processing of coral remnants is particularly relevant (see www.naturesbenefit.com). Furthermore, these issues are of great relevance to the ecology. Coral reefs are threatened and any collection process that threatens survival of the coral reefs must be avoided (www.coralcalciuminformation.com).

Coral reefs are a very important focus of marine life. I reiterate that a any one time, a large proportion of sea dwelling organisms visit temperate waters where coral reefs are found. The coral reefs have their own rich array of inhabitants. With the popularization of coral calcium as a food supplement and increasing pressure to harvest coral remnants from the sea (and from land adjacent to water), the whole issue of environmental protection for the Rukuyuku Islands must become a concern. Fortunately, the environment in Okinawa has been well-policed by the Japanese Government. At present, no damage to coral reefs around Okinawa, Japan has been observed or reported, despite increased collection of coral sand.

COLLECTION AND PROCESSING CORAL

I have attempted, with great intensity of effort, to contact many suppliers of coral material from Okinawa and request information about coral processing techniques, coral collection and measured compositions of various commercial forms of coral calcium products (marine coral minerals or fossilized stony coral minerals). Whilst there appear to be many types of commercially available coral from Okinawa, these apparent "different" types of "commercial coral calcium or sand" are a function of the number of different companies supplying coral, rather than different sources of the base materials of the crude coral remnants (the "coral sand"). These coral remnants (coral sand) are used to produce the finished, coral calcium, dietary supplement.

Clearly, the best research on coral production may done by visiting the many processing facilities or collection points in Okinawa where direct observations of the various processing techniques could be observed. However, the commercial production of coral calcium involves several well kept secrets. It sounds simple, but the "processors of coral" closely guard their business practice. This circumstance has arisen largely because coral calcium is now a valuable commodity which is at the root of a competitive business environment, especially in the US.

The Japanese government has taken steps to regulate the harvesting of coral which comes from two basic sources. The first source is land-based collection (mining) and the second is sea- based collection (suction collections from ocean beds). I stress that my opinion is that all coral remnants (dead corals) are fossils. They are essentially dead pieces of coral that fall from the reef as a consequence of environmental influences e.g. underwater currents, coral "munching" by marine life etc. The reefs have been present in Okinawa for eons and fossilized coral litters the ocean floor for miles around the reef.

As coral calcium becomes more popular, "trade secrets" start to emerge. Whilst obtaining information from suppliers is one thing, I had to find a way to investigate matters further by obtaining reliable, collateral information from people who had visited facilities in Okinawa, where coral is processed and collected. At the time of writing, I was told that only one of the two acclaimed North American experts, and independent authors of books on the subject of coral calcium, had visited Okinawa. This expert is Dr. Bruce Halstead MD.

INFORMED OPINION ON
CORAL COLLECTION AND HANDLING

I have had the pleasure and opportunity to have a detailed interview with Mr. Andy Bowers, an executive from the company Coral, Inc. of Nevada; and receive information from several other individuals who have a detailed knowledge of the oceans around Okinawa. The information obtained from Mr. Bowers complemented my own direct research with Okinawan suppliers of coral material. Mr. A. Bowers visited many coral processing facilities in Okinawa in the early part of 2002. His visit to Okinawa, Japan clarified my own sleuthing on the subject. I have studied all available specifications of all commercial forms of coral calcium (at least those about which I could obtain credible information). There are companies with "exclusive" supply arrangements who do not discuss matters in an open manner.

To summarize my own analysis of the situation, the overall picture of commercial coral calcium is confusing or it is perhaps purposely confused? There are companies who supply coral sand products only (collection operations), some who process it and many more who broker or sell finished coral calcium remnants, in both Japan and the USA. A couple of Japanese companies that supply coral calcium appear to be vertically integrated, albeit through different corporate identities. Each company has variable support from research scientists and variable frequency of analyses of each coral product batch. There appears to be some inconsistency in processing and some other "production matters" are hard to define or believe.

Whilst a number of sales and processing companies (about a dozen key companies) exist in Okinawa, it has been observed allegedly that below-sea coral generally comes from only one commercial collection operation. Again, this matter is "hotly debated". Concerning below-sea coral calcium, Mr. Bowers states "the processors are different than the collectors, the processors do not own the boats and, therefore, most companies (producing coral calcium from below-sea collected coral sand) start with the same raw material that is suctioned from the ocean floor". There are several Japanese suppliers who contradict Mr. Bowers.

To test this situation Mr. Bowers collected raw material (unprocessed coral) from more than one source and confirmed its characteristics to be the same. In other words, different processing companies were using the same coral remnants from a presumed similar collection point in the ocean. However, there are claims that this is not the case – the facts are somewhat elusive, but they may be explained (see section on blended coral processing). I have examined crude coral sand sent directly from Okinawa and I have specifications sharing magnesium contents from less than 1% to more than 10% with calcium contents between 25% and 35%, approximately.

Contrary to other uninformed assertions, the coral sand is collected often a long distance (more than one or two miles) away from the actual reef, using an underwater suction apparatus (rather like a giant "Hoover"). Observers have commented on the results of this ocean- floor-suctioning process used to collect coral. Mr. Bowers believes that the collection process is quite disturbing to the seabed. Mr. Bowers stated that "a lot of underwater plant material is disturbed in the collection process". Again, others disagree.

These direct observations do not confirm the notions expressed by other authors on the subject of coral calcium (or pundits or several US internet sales operations of coral calcium). In contrast, it has been reported by others that coral remnants are removed from locations that enhance the growth or coral reefs. They argue that coral sand chokes the reefs and stunts its growth. This is probably a mere speculation (or "fairy tale"). Whilst these opinions do question to some degree the ecological consequences of the harvesting of coral sand, the Japanese Government and the producers assert that there are no environmental problems present or anticipated.

TYPES OF CORAL AND PROCESSING

Having determined that there are two basic forms of "fossilized" coral predominantly (land-based or sea-based) an obvious question arises. "Which type is the best type?" Predictably the answer to this question is not simple. Many ill informed opinions have been expressed on "the best form of coral" and this has caused massive confusion, especially among consumers of potentially valuable coral calcium supplements. Contrary to popular misconceptions, the best type of coral material is not necessarily derived from ocean based or land-based coral sand deposits. There is both good and bas types of land-based or sea-based coral sand or coral remnants. The real answer to this question on the best types of coral is that each type may have different advantages and potential disadvantages and appropriate selections must be made based on informed opinions (see www.naturesbenefit.com). The quest for knowledge to give a consumer an informed opinion about coral calcium supplements is the principal reason why I wrote this book.

The "widely-perceived" advantage of below-sea collected coral has been related to its enhanced magnesium content, in comparison to the magnesium content of land-based coral. This issue could be a "fairy tale". However, land based coral may have a slightly greater calcium content per weight than some below-sea coral, at least in its finished format as coral calcium. Arguably, land based coral tends to have superior characteristics because of its calcium content, especially if the "calcium factor" is the principal focus of health interests. Again, I stress that the health benefits of coral calcium (marine coral minerals or fossilized stony coral minerals) is much more than a function of its general mineral content than its content of "calcium alone".

It has been stated incorrectly that Japanese consumers of coral judge the quality of coral by its natural magnesium content. This is not an issue of "quality" and such distinctions do not figure in the Okinawans person's mind or in the mind of "clinicians" who have used "coral calcium treatments". It is more an issue of expense of collection and processing, where certain types of high- magnesium-containing marine coral (or blended marine coral) require a more cumbersome and intensive collection and processing technique (vide infra). Thus, it is the processors who judge coral by its magnesium content, not the users.

I stress that my comments refer to only "certain types" of below-sea coral minerals because there are relatively inexpensive forms of marine coral available which are not "processed" to remove heavy metals, such as lead and mercury. Thus, certain types of marine coral are vastly "inferior" to other types of marine coral and clearly inferior to land based coral because of their potential content of heavy metals. This type of below-sea collected coral with inferior characteristics may be being used in some supplements in the US, according to suppliers.

INFERIOR CORAL CALCIUM

Whilst the word "inferior" operates in describing some inferior forms of sea-collected coral sand, better words may be potentially "dangerous" because this "unprocessed" cruder form of below-sea collected coral has a higher lead content (or toxic heavy metal content) than other forms of coral calcium. Furthermore, it does not conform to US government regulations, such as proposition in 65 in the State of California. This inferior form of coral should be excluded from supplements in the US. For these reasons, I restrict a lot of my statements on coral calcium use to forms of coral calcium supplements that are collected and processed in an appropriate manner (www.naturesbenefit.com). My recommendations are based upon disclosures by manufacturers of coral calcium, concerning issues that determine safety. Only those products where there is a documented health benefit of their use are recommended, even though some documentation of health benefits may be anecdotal. When it comes to purchasing a coral calcium supplement, the adage "caveat empeator" must apply. Well processed, high grade coral is not cheap! Beware, discounted coral calcium!

The form of below-sea collected coral that is safe and preferred is treated and screened for its heavy metal content, especially lead and mercury (www.naturesbenefit.com). This form of coral is available in different grain sizes (www.naturesbenefit.com). It is predictably an expensive form of coral and it is balanced with calcium and magnesium in a 2:1 ratio. When processors are asked about the collection and nature of this type of coral, they do not (or will not) describe the exact treatment for heavy metal exclusion. Some observers indicate (or speculate?) that the heavy metals are removed sometimes by the application of intense heat (heating up to 1000 degrees Celsius). At these temperatures, coral calcium will oxidize (calcinate), but high grade coral is not calcinated (www.naturesbenefit.com)

As previously stated, marine coral has been preferred by some because of its alleged higher, "natural" magnesium content. Elements may leach out of land-coral over years, but land based coral can still be shown by analysis to contain up to 74 trace elements. Whilst I believe that elements can "leach out "of land-based coral, why would only magnesium be leached? The professed advantage of underwater coral is its apparent two to one balance of calcium to magnesium (alleged by some to be natural). Laboratory analysis of "processed" marine coral shows a variable calcium content (no less than 24%) with a relatively high magnesium content (no less than 11%). Whilst this ratio is stated by the suppliers to be a natural occurrence, some individuals doubt this representation that is or has been made to US consumers.

"BLENDED CORAL"

Several people doubt the existence of "perfect" coral sand, as defined by a "naturally occurring", 2 to 1 calcium to magnesium balance. Suppliers have stated that there is a specific location where this type of naturally occurring, 2 to 1, calcium to magnesium, balanced coral exists. I have requested certification of this fact from suppliers and in many cases the question remained unanswered; and, in one case, I was promised an affidavit from a Japanese Scientist concerning the natural deposits of coral sand containing calcium and magnesium in a "perfect" 2:1 balance, but I am still waiting. However, in September 2002, I was sent samples and specifications on three unprocessed, coral sand samples that seemed to imply that it has approximately 11% magnesium content. This high magnesium content was attributed by the supplier to be related to a specific, but secret, underwater collection point; but others stated that blending of "naturally" high magnesium types of below-sea coral occurs during processing. It is my belief that magnesium is added, until I can prove otherwise.

For more than one year, I have repeatedly questioned suppliers about he magnesium content of coral calcium. It appears that there is coral sand (the precursor of the supplement coral calcium) with a high magnesium content, but I doubt the occurrence of a form of coral remnants with a perfect balance of calcium to magnesium of 2 to 1. It seems (according to some sources) that the below-sea coral used in supplements is created by a blend of coral material collected from the ocean floor using coral sand of variable magnesium content. This form of blended coral calcium is high quality, bioactive marine material that represents an excellent holistic source of minerals. It is used in only a couple or more of the leading brands of coral calcium supplements and it is a highly recommended form of below-sea collected coral sand (Barefoot Coral Calcium Plus™, Marine coral Minerals™ Natures Benefit Inc. of Newark, NJ, www.naturesbenefit.com).

THE IMPERFECT WORLD OF CORAL CALCIUM

By now, one can see that the world of coral collection and processing is not ideal and it is highly complex. Turning attention to land based coral, one can now make a case that this form may be highly desirable for use as a food or dietary supplement, a least in terms of its calcium content and perhaps it significance to the environment. This opinion is strongly espoused by Dr. Bruce Halstead MD who commands a respected opinion given his background, training and contributions to marine medical science. Land-based coral contains up to about 40% calcium (35 - 37.5% in recent analyses), but its magnesium content is often less than 1%. Please note, the sand applies to many types of marine coral, especially the types used in tea bags. Consumers must recognize that much coral sand collected below-sea level has a similar, relatively low, magnesium content. This lower content of magnesium can easily be compensated for by adding a suitable magnesium source (e.g. oxide or carbonate). Whilst this practice has been criticized by some as not "natural", there is no evidence that magnesium supplemented (or "unsupple-

mented") coral is inferior in its medical benefits to otherwise
"alleged", naturally-blended 2:1 (calcium to magnesium) forms of
coral calcium. Again, I stress that the perfect 2:1 balance of calcium
to magnesium in coral sand may not occur in nature?

I restate that claims that below-sea derived coral calcium is
more effective for health than land based coral calcium CANNOT
BE SUBSTANTIATED. In fact, it is argued that most published testimonials in the US may have come from land based coral use in
supplements or even the use of water treated with coral enclosed in
tea bags (also land-based coral). Therefore the issue "Which is
best? Land or under-the-sea-level coral material?" - remains the
subject of debate and a lot of uninformed rhetoric. Both forms of
coral calcium, precursor material (land or below-sea collected) have
been associated with claims of major health benefit. Table 1 starts
to summarize some of the issues (matters of fact) related to different types of coral.

Below-Sea Coral Calcium	Land-Based Coral Calcium
Some types quite "Low" in calcium	Up to 38% calcium, +/- 20%
Higher magnesium (added or blended?)	Magnesium easily and appropriately added, but not definitely required
Ecological concern, but no damage reported.	Less concern about environmental consequences
More heavy metals and p ollutants in untreated forms	Less toxic metal contamination
Processed with heat sometimes	Processed often with ozone, With heat
Health benefits described (anecdotal)	Health benefits described (anecdotal)

**Table 1: Exploring some of the pro's and con's of marine and land based
coral calcium. Note, both types have been used in capsules, powders
and "tea bags".**

OPTIMIZING CORAL CALCIUM USE

Perhaps, more important than discussions about sources of coral calcium in Okinawa, Japan (and its processing) are questions relating to the beneficial outcome of taking specific forms of coral calcium. These issues become "very muddy" when different types of coral calcium supplements are considered. There are few scientific studies of their use as nutritional "treatment" and "testimonials" of benefit used to support the coral calcium product in question do not always specify which kind of coral is being used by the reported beneficiary. Two diametrically opposing opinions have surfaced in the language of marketing coral calcium. In brief, Mr. R. Barefoot prefers below-sea coral, but states "all coral is fantastic", and Dr. Bruce Halstead MD (the eminent physician, marine biologist and biomedical expert on marine organisms) prefers land-based stony coral minerals for use in nutraceuticals (see www.naturesbenefit.com).

There are varying sources of testimonials, using below-sea and above ground coral calcium taken in capsules, powders and even coral calcium "tea bag" treated water. I am personally aware of hundreds of people who have claimed benefit. Whilst it is sometimes argued that testimonials are not "cast-iron-proof" of benefit one must be impressed by the sheer volume and consistency of supportive testimonials that have appeared in books, articles, "chat rooms" on the Internet and on the many web pages on the internet. Users of coral calcium are "voting with dollars" by re-ordering coral calcium as a consequence of their perceived health benefits from this dietary supplement.

A compilation of testimonials is present in Mr. Barefoot's book "Barefoot on Coral Calcium" (www.wellnesspublishing.com), but some of these testimonials may have been as a result of people taking coral calcium water derived from teabag enclosed coral, some may be from land-based coral and some allegedly from below-sea coral, at least according to several dietary supplement companies.

SOME COMPANIES LEAD THE WAY

Accepting (with residual arguments) that there may be some benefits to be derived from a higher magnesium content or a different micronutrient profile of below- sea coral (both misnamed coral calcium), there emerges a clear justification for the use of high quality below-sea collected coral calcium and high quality land-collected coral. I stress, high quality (www.naturesbenefit.com, see the book "Barefoot on Coral Calcium" by R. barefoot and the book "Fossil Stony Coral Minerals and Their Nutritional Application" by B. Halstead MD, at www.wellnesspublishing.com).

For these and other reasons stated earlier, Natures Benefit Inc. have created four different types of coral calcium supplements. Natures Benefit Inc. believes that it now is important to define the types of coral used in dietary supplements. This company has evolved to use two different forms of coral in its four products. Two of the products contain high grade marine-collected coral calcium. (Barefoot Coral Calcium Plus™ or Barefoot Coral Calcium Formula and Marine Coral Minerals™). These products contain marine collected coral in a newly recommended daily dose of 1.5 grams per day in three capsules. The remaining two products contain land-collected coral calcium in a newly recommended daily dose of 1.5 grams per day in capsules (Halstead Coral Calcium™) or 3 grams per day in plain powder (Coral Calcium Powder™). These products are encapsulated fossilized, stony minerals called Halstead Coral Calcium™ (1.5g/day) or 100% Pure Coral Calcium Powder™ (see www.naturesbenefit.com). Unlike most other companies, Natures Benefit Inc. have published specifications with full disclosure on the internet.

HOW TO TAKE CORAL

Coral calcium is consumed in dietary supplements in the form of powders, capsules of different types (www.naturesbenefit.com) or by drinking coral water, prepared by placing coral enclosed teabags in drinking waters. Factors such as convenience, beliefs and nutritional intentions enter arguments about which is the best form of coral to take. Aside from these considerations, one must examine how coral calcium is used in traditional settings, such as those in Okinawa, Japan. Traditionally, coral has been used as a certified food grade supplement (Certified first in July 1989 by the Japanese Government) in a powder form in food preparation. Processed or fermented soy products such as tofu can be "set" during preparation by the addition of coral calcium powder. This "firm-type" of tofu combines the health benefits of soy with calcium and mineral enrichment. Calcium combined with soy protein has many potential health benefits including the nutritional support of bone health and cardiovascular health (see Holt S. The Soy Revolution, Dell Publishing, Random House, 1999, available at www.wellnesspublishing.com).

Whilst focused accounts of the health benefits of coral calcium for the people of Okinawa, Japan people stress "coral" as health-giving, I reiterate that other factors operate to promote health in the population. The diet of the average Okinawan is very different from a Standard American Diet (SAD). It is higher in fiber, essential fatty acids (omega-3 fatty acids), vegetable-protein, fruit and vegetables and much lower in saturated fat, simple sugar and cholesterol intake. However, more salt may be present in the Okinawan diet – a negative issue that may be linked to the cause of increased problems with gastric cancer and stroke in Japanese people.

I have reviewed the role of soy in promoting health in Asian communities in my two books (Holt S, "Soya for Health", Mary Ann Liebert publishers Inc, Larchmont, NY, 1994 and Holt S, "The Soy Revolution" Dell Publishing, Random House, NY, NY, 1999). The soy intake of Okinawans has peaked in recent years and it may be declining. I believe that soy in the diet of Okinawans contributes to their health and well-being. There is a tradition of eating pork in Okinawa often prepared in the regional dish called "Champuru" – a stir fried dish of vegetables, tofu and pork. A discussion of dietary habits in Okinawa is relevant because the basis of some claims of the health benefits of coral calcium come from the observations of relative good health and longevity that is determined by the lifestyle of Okinawan people.

It is logical to reason that "whole coral calcium" in powder or pills (below-sea level collected coral minerals or fossilized stony coral minerals) are the best ways to take coral calcium as a supplement. Capsules or powders of coral calcium seem ideal and convenient when swallowed whole, added to food or taken by emptying capsules (for the "so-inclined") into beverages or on food. Whilst I do not ignore that coral tea bags, providing coral water, have been associated with reported (anecdotal) health benefits, coral calcium is relatively insoluble and only a small percentage of the coral minerals dissolve the "coral water". Thus, coral treated water delivers only very small amounts of minerals and elements for absorption into the body. Thus, the majority opinion is that coral is best consumed in capsules with good dissolution characteristics to present the whole coral for digestion and absorption in the gastrointestinal tract.

Later in this book, I discuss the "cell salt theory" or "Schuessler's Theory" (an extension of homeopathic medicine) of health maintenance. These hypotheses may provide support for the use of coral water produced from tea-bag enclosed coral. The "cell salt theory" is described in much greater detail later in this book, as I attempt to examine how coral calcium may work to cause a health benefit.

HOW MUCH CORAL SHOULD BE TAKEN?

The optimal daily dose of coral calcium (marine coral minerals or fossilized stony coral minerals) is a best guess. The answer to this question about the recommended daily intake of coral calcium is not only unknown, it is not simple. We have a confusing precedent upon which we can start to address the issue of ideal doses of coral calcium in supplements. First, the traditional use of coral calcium involves intake of at least gram amounts or greater daily. However, one may not dismiss the reports that coral water, containing only small amounts of dissolved coral minerals, may be beneficial for health. This enigma may be related to the knowledge that only small amounts of minerals (cell salts) may have beneficial effects (e.g. a homeopathic effect, or the "Schuessler effect" – see later). Homeopathy is a treatment science where infinitesimal amounts of various natural substances are believed to have treatment properties.

In general, good responses have been reported (anecdotal) with daily intakes of 1 gram (1000 mg of coral) of

marine or land-based coral with or without the addition of magnesium. However, given the precedent for higher intakes of coral in traditional settings, I believe that at least 1.5 g. of coral calcium of either type (land or sea collected coral calcium), may be more optimal. I have revised my recommendations to 1.5 grams per day of coral calcium in three capsules, based on this reasoning.

It could be argued that the higher the concentration of calcium taken from coral the better, up to an arbitrarily recommended maximum of 2 grams per day of elemental calcium, where indicated and safe. Now comes an issue that may surprise the consumer. The current recommended daily amounts of intake of coral calcium by the majority of supplement companies do not meet the recommended daily intakes (RDI) of calcium that are considered by most nutritional scientists to be optimal. A little simple arithmetic will help to explain this important issue and reinforce my recommendation of increasing the amount of coral calcium intake to 1.5 grams per day. Even though calcium from coral calcium is well-absorbed in comparison to several other forms of calcium supplements, the amount of calcium delivered in most coral products is well below recommended daily intakes, another reason why I recommend at least 1.5 g/day (www.naturesbenefit.com).

CALCIUM CONTENT OF CORAL CALCIUM

High quality, below-sea collected coral contains about 25 to 38% calcium, so only 240 – 380 mg or more of elemental calcium is available from a dose of 1000mg (1 gram) of coral calcium. To supply a recommended daily intake of calcium of 1000 mg (RDI 100%), one would have to take about 3 - 4 grams of this type of marine coral. Since average daily doses of coral calcium in most coral calcium products are recommended at 1000 mg in two capsules, to take the recommended daily intake (RDI) of calcium (assuming it to be 1000 mg per day) would require the taking of at least four <u>standard coral calcium capsules!</u> Even land collected coral with its variably higher calcium content still does not meet the expectations of standard, common (RDI) recommended daily intake in generally recommended dosages.

For these reasons, I stress that people who take coral calcium must still consider the importance of sticking with a calcium-rich diet. I have found that the understanding of calcium intake with coral is the single most confusing issue for consumers of coral calcium. On a practical level, I advise patients who are looking for optimal calcium intake (at the higher levels of RDI) that they should take a diet that provides at least 500mg of elemental calcium and try to supplement about 1000mg of elemental calcium from other sources such as coral calcium combined with other calcium supplements if necessary (see www.naturesbenefit, www.miracal.com, www.antiporosis.com). What I am describing is an "eye-opener" for many consumers, but it is matter of fact. The issues will become even clearer as I discuss the general issues of calcium supplementation, later in this book. The focus on the calcium factor alone is a limited perspective.

OPTIMIZING THE CORAL CALCIUM SUPPLEMENT

Based on the information available and accepting its occasional limitations, my clear recommendations for an ideal coral calcium supplement emerge from the following:

The calcium content of the coral is important. In this respect, some land-based coral may be preferred over below-sea collected coral calcium because of its relatively high calcium content. Regardless of whether or not coral collected from above or below-sea level is used as a supplement, I see some advantages in adding extra sources of elemental calcium in the diet, if an RDI of 1000 mg (or greater) of calcium is desired (see section on egg shell calcium or www.miracal.com).

Marine coral has some putative advantages, providing that high quality, lead-free, pollutant-free coral is used (see-land and below-sea collected coral calcium, Barefoot Coral Calcium™, Halstead Coral Calcium™, Coral Calcium Powder™ and Marine Coral Minerals™, www.naturesbenefit.com). Coral collected from the ocean floor should only be used if it can be certified free of heavy metals or other contaminants. There is marine or below-sea-collected coral available in some supplements that contains unacceptable levels of lead and this form of coral is not approved for sale in the US, at least according to California State legislation, otherwise called Proposition 65 (www.coralcalciuminformation.com).

Coral calcium alone may not supply all required calcium for most people in current common recommended daily intakes of 1g/day or greater. A dose of 1.5 grams per day of coral calcium is more desirable (www.naturesbenefit.com).

Nature's imprint for the correct assimilation of calcium by the body is believed, arguably, to be calcium to magnesium balanced in a ratio of two parts calcium to one part magnesium. This point is arguable and benefit has been described with "coral calcium" that has a lower magnesium content (see book by B. W. Halstead MD entitled "Fossil Stony Coral Minerals and Their Nutritional Application", 1999).

The nutritional benefits of coral calcium may, or may not, be enhanced by the addition of co-factors such as vitamins and other specific trace elements that have a clear biological role in supporting body structures and functions (see Barefoot Coral Calcium™, www.naturesbenefit.com). Excessive doses of fat soluble vitamins (e.g. vitamin D, A and K) should be avoided, as should toxic metals, e.g. cesium.

Coral calcium supplements must use material that is free from toxic metals and organic pollutants found in the ocean (e.g. lead, mercury, cadmium, PCB's - see www.naturesbenefit.com) or added to supplements e.g. cesium.

Coral calcium supplements should contain coral material for which there is a clear precedent of benefit. This benefit is described at least equally with land based and below-sea level coral calcium (see the work of Mr. Barefoot or that of Dr. B Halstead MD at www.well-nesspublishing.com).

In terms of effectiveness, land based and below-sea level coral appear to be equivalent in described benefits, but many of these benefits are anecdotal descriptions.

Only coral remnants that are collected with due attention to the support of the environment should be used in coral calcium supplements, regardless of whether or not they are collected from land or sea (www.naturesbenefit.com).

On the basis of the above statements, I propose what I believe to be optimum formulas for coral calcium supplements. My formulas differ from the common recommendations, notably by my recommendation of at a least 1.5gm of whole coral calcium under-water-based (Barefoot Coral Calcium or Marine Coral Minerals™ www.naturesbenefit.com) or land-based coral calcium (Halstead "Coral Calcium™ or Coral Calcium Powder™, www.naturesbenefit.com). I stress that high quality land and below-sea collected coral are both potentially beneficial supplements.

Some manufacturers avoid the extra amounts of coral calcium in their supplements, because higher doses of coral calcium obviously increases the cost of the product (by at least 30%) and this takes margins out of their sales. I support a co-administration of vitamin E, D, A and C with coral calcium in some cases for their obvious health benefits and this type of formulation is found in Barefoot Coral Calcium Plus™ (www.naturesbenefit.com). Vitamin D is essential for calcium absorption and utilization in the body, but high dosages must be avoided. Further, I recommend in some formulations the addition of certain micronutrient metals which have a well-defined role in health, notably selenium, zinc, boron, chromium and molybdenum. I do not support the use of metals or elements such as cesium, nickel or silver in coral formulations. How important it is to present the coral calcium, in a balance of calcium to magnesium of two parts calcium to one part magnesium, remains debatable, but it is available in Barefoots Coral Calcium Plus™ and Marine Coral Minerals™ in doses of 1.5 grams per day.

Concerning specific coral content, I recommend both land-collected and below-sea-collected coral for the many of reasons defined earlier. Consumers must be given choices. My recommendations have been developed by a combination of feedback on reported individual benefits, studied necessarily in an uncontrolled manner, and my own reasoning that has been applied to what is known to be factual about coral calcium supplements. The formulas that I recommend are described in table 2 as supplement facts panels. In these coral calcium products, at least 1.5 grams of high quality coral calcium are recommended on a daily basis. These products deliver more coral than most other brands, at the time of writing.

Marine Coral Minerals™:
Servings per container: 30, Serving Size: 3 capsules contain:

100% High Grade Coral Calcium from Okinawa Japan	1500 mg
Calcium (26% RDI)	360 mg
Magnesium (45% RDI) from coral magnesium carbonate	180 mg

With trace minerals with natural variability including: selenium, zinc, Copper, potassium, iodize, iron and up to 70 other mineral elements all in parts per million Other ingredients: Silicon dioxide, cellulose, magnesium steorate and gelatin. No cholesterol, fat and calories.

Coral Calcium Powder™:
Servings per container: 30, Serving Size: 3 g (one scoop) contains:

	Amount Per Serving	% Daily Value
High Grade Coral Calcium	3 g	N/A
Calcium (from coral)	1200 mg	120%
Magnesium (from coral)	30 mg	7.5%

Halstead Stony Coral Minerals Coral Calcium™:
Servings per container: 30, Serving Seize 3
capsules contain:

	Amount Per Serving	% Daily Value
Stony Coral Minerals	1500 mg	N/A
Calcium from Coral Calcium	600 mg	60%
Magnesium from Coral Calcium	15 mg	3.5%

Barefoot Coral Calcium Plus™:
Servings per container: 30, Serving Size 3 capsules contain:

	Amount Per Serving	% Daily Value
Coral Calcium (up to 70 trace minerals and elements with natural variability)	1500 mg	
Vitamin C (as Ascorbic Acid)	60 mg	100%
Vitamin D3 (as Cholecalciferol)	400 IU	100%
Vitamin E (natural)	30 IU	100%
Vitamin A	2197 IU	44%
Calcium (from coral calcium)	380 mg	36%
Iodine (Kelp)	10 mcg	7%
Magnesium (from Coral Calcium)	180 mg	45%
Zinc (as Zinc Oxide)	15 mg	100%
Selenium (as amino acid chelate)	20 mcg	29%
Copper (as amino acid chelate)	30 mcg	2%
Manganese (as amino acid chelate)	0 mcg	<1%
Chromium (as amino acid chelate)	120 mcg	100%
Molybdenum (as amino acid chelate)	10 mcg	13%
Vanadium (as amino acid chelate)	30 mcg	*
Boron (as amino acid chelate)	20 mcg	*

* Daily Value not established / Natural Calcium:Magnesium Ratio

Table 2: This table describes the supplements facts panels on some of the leading brands of coral calcium that are sold in the United States. Information was supplied with the permission of Natures Benefit Inc. www.naturesbenefit.com.

READING LABELS

I display the formulas in a typical supplement facts panel in table 2 to help consumers understand how to interpret the average, coral calcium, dietary supplement label. Readers should please note that the amount of calcium listed on the supplement facts label (legal requirements) differs from the total amount of coral in the product. This is simply because coral calcium is <u>much more than just calcium.</u> It is a mixture of coral debris (ash) containing other minerals and elements elaborated by the living coral. Analyses of coral show up to 74 different micromineral associated elements. Again, I stress the misleading nature of the name "coral calcium" and that is why I have preferred on occasion to call coral calcium by several, interchangeable names including "marine coral minerals", "stony coral minerals", "fossilized coral minerals" and "coral remnants".

MORE ABOUT THE COMBINING OF NUTRIENTS WITH CORAL

The use of combined formulas of coral calcium with other vitamins and elements is very popular, but many people already take multivitamins or other supplements, such that they are better suited to taking the coral calcium alone. For this circumstance, I recommend products that have no vitamin additives (e.g. Marine Coral Minerals™, Halstead Coral Calcium™ and Coral Calcium Powder™). These coral calcium products are all 100% pure coral calcium in capsules without vitamin additives. Coral Calcium Powder™ is pure coral powder taken with a scoop and added to food or water, in a dose of up to 3 g/day. This form of coral calcium supplement is similar in its delivery with the traditional use of coral calcium food supplements in Japan. Excessive intake of vitamin D, vitamin A and vitamin K are to be avoided. Vitamin K has been added to some coral calcium supplements, but I consider this to be unnecessary because most requirement are met for vitamin K by its synthesis on the large bowel and its intake in the average diet. Furthermore, vitamin K affects blood clotting and excessive supplementation could increase risks of bleeding, especially in people receiving blood-thinning medications.

HOW DOES CORAL WORK: STARTING WITH MINERAL DEPLETION

I fear that this book has started to appear to pose more questions than answers. It should come as no surprise, when I now state that much speculation exists on how coral calcium may exert a health benefit. It is clear that many elements and minerals are necessary for the support of vital body structures and functions. Enzyme systems in the body which help to control the chemistry of life often require specific elements as co-factors, in order that they can operate efficiently. A co-factor in the chemistry of life can be a metal or a vitamin. For example, calcium exerts effects on many body functions including how muscles contract, how the heart beats and even how messages are transmitted to cells. These actions of calcium permit the body to function in a normal manner. The same is true of many other elements or minerals e.g. magnesium, zinc, selenium etc.

Chemical analyses of many types of coral calcium show that it contains up to 74 different elements derived from the earth's crust and elaborated originally by live coral polyps from sea water. If one examines the mineral content of the human body, one finds that all minerals that occur in nature are present to variable degrees. Calcium is a dominant element in the body of many living organisms, but it is not the only important nutrient mineral. The importance of mineral supplementation has been magnified by reports that mineral deficiencies in Western Society may be much more common than people realize. Evidence has emerged that our immediate environment may be considered to be "depleted" of minerals and certain key elements.

Much agricultural land has been farmed extensively and a number of nutrient deficiencies in soils are described. Since plants derive their composition from the soil, factors such as mineral deficiency may lead to a lower nutrient value of some fruits and vegetables. Further, several types of mineral or elemental deficiency lead to certain acute and chronic diseases in humans. For example, this metal deficiency has been associated with poor immune function and zinc is necessary for the function of the hormone insulin. Insulin function is a major issue for public health, given the occurrence of the metabolic syndrome X in up to 70 million

American people (see Holt S, Combat Syndrome X, Y and Z...,
www.wellnesspublishing.com).

There are many other examples of how elements (available
as minerals) promote well-being e.g. boron for bone health, magnesium for cardiovascular function, chromium for insulin function,
etc. However, the amount of many micronutrient metals found in
coral calcium is quite small. The small concentrations of many
minerals in "coral calcium" does not defeat all arguments in favor
of the potential effectiveness of coral calcium for health. Indeed, the
"cell salt theory" which is an extension of homeopathic medicine
(Schuessler's Theory) provides support for the claims of health benefits of "small" concentrations of supplemented minerals.
Schuessler's Theory is based on "biochemic principals", but these
"theories" have not been embraced by all physicians (vide infra).

MINERAL REQUIREMENTS ARE DEBATED

The optimal amount of intake of various minerals that one
requires in a healthy diet has been subject to much debate. Many
contemporary nutritionists feel that recommended daily intake
(RDI) of certain vitamins or minerals are insufficient for many people. Authors of popular books on the subject of vitamin and mineral supplements stress that recommended daily allowances (or
recommended daily intakes) of vital nutrients are designed only to
prevent deficiencies of nutrients. Conventional recommendations
for "healthy" mineral intake have been subject to continuing revi-
sion. Certainly, recommended daily intakes of calcium for health
have been increased over the past few years.

Shari Lieberman PhD and Nancy Bruning (authors of the
book entitled "The Real Vitamin & Mineral Book") have proposed
that not all nutrients can be obtained from today's regular food supplies. These authors stress that recommended daily intakes (RDI)
of minerals vary considerably among individuals and that current
recommended mineral intake may not guarantee optimal health.
Further, these authors imply that extensive food tables which
describe the nutrient value of certain foods tend to overestimate
nutrient contents of many foods. The analogy used by Dr.
Lieberman and Ms Bruning is that "like clothes" (referring to recommended daily intakes of minerals, RDI) do not conform to the

idea that "one size fits all". Despite the arguments, it is clear in scientific literature that certain vitamins and minerals afford protection against the development of disease; and in some cases they many even counteract the effect of environmental pollution on health.

MORE OR LESS MINERALS?

Many nutritionists claim that there is widespread micronutrient deficiency in the population, especially specific types of trace elements or minerals. However, one must not be too quick to assume that more is necessarily better, especially when it comes to vitamins and minerals. There are many experiments that show that excess amounts of certain minerals do not have a better effect on health than smaller amounts of intake. Moreover, some essential micronutrients and elements are toxic when given in excess. Thus, the proponents of excessive mineral intake for health have to be questioned. For example, selenium which is recommended for its indirect antioxidant effects, and other benefits on health, can cause cardiovascular problems when taken in very high doses. In contrast, selenium in modest amounts can benefit cardiovascular health.

In general, high doses of water soluble vitamins, such as vitamin C (up to 5g/day, an amount much greater than RDI) are believed by many physicians to be relatively harmless. However, very high concentrations of vitamin C (greater than 5 grams per day) when given alone may have a negative health effect, by promoting, rather than preventing, oxidative stress in the body. The toxicity of fat soluble vitamins in high dosages is not in question. More than the recommended daily intake of vitamin D, in the absence of vitamin D deficiency, cannot be considered health giving. In this regard, I disagree with recommendations for liberal vitamin D intake, unless it is supervised by a knowledgeable healthcare giver. In addition, excessive intake of vitamins A and K can have quite serious consequences. The consensus opinion in medicine is that large doses of fat soluble vitamins are to be avoided (vitamins A, D, E and K), except under special medical circumstances, where close supervision must occur.

I cannot question the proposal that mineral intake from coral calcium would be beneficial for many people who may be missing important elements in their diet. Certainly, the micronutrient content of commonly-eaten, processed food is constantly in question. Further, agricultural practices that are used to increase crop yields have been blamed as an indirect cause of nutrient deficiency in the population. A large proportion of the population have turned to fast food or junk food as a staple component of their diet. These circumstances may help foster widespread micronutrient (mineral) deficiency in modern society.

MINERAL SALTS AND HEALTH

Coral calcium (marine or stony coral minerals etc.) appear to be an attractive mineral supplement to many people, but this supplement may not necessarily exert its actions by the direct supply of commonly recommended amounts of certain nutrients (especially RDI). This reasoning applies to situations where "desired" amounts of minerals are defined as widely accepted, recommended daily intakes (RDI). I have suggested previously that coral calcium may work by a homeopathic mechanism.

This proposal may explain why people drinking coral water, which contains very tiny amounts of many minerals, could have the benefits that have been described in some testimonials. Coral calcium only dissolves in very small amounts in water and coral calcium, in turn, contains only very small amounts of many minerals. Is coral water a homeopathic remedy?

Homeopathy is a medical specialty where very small doses of natural agents are use to treat a variety of diseases. A basic principle of homeopathic medicine is the use of "like to treat like" and inorganic material is used in various types of homeopathy. One common form of homeopathy is called "lithotherapy", where dilutions of natural minerals or "rocks" (e.g. coral) are used in treatment. Is the drinking of coral water a form of homeopathic lithotherapy?

I stress that very tiny amounts of minerals are present in homeopathic treatments. Lithotherapy is an extension of homeopathic treatments that have been used in Germany and other

Western countries for many years. This type of therapy has been
expanded by some researchers and referred to as cell salt therapy,
as originally proposed by Dr. W. Schuessler MD. Dr. Schuessler was
a German physician who developed the "biochemic" extensions of
homeopathic medicine. There have been modern accounts of the
success of cell salt therapy and some extensions of this therapy have
included the administration of a variety of minerals or elements in
trace amounts. If a homeopathic effect of coral calcium occurs, the
distinction between the relative benefits of different types of coral
calcium supplements (capsules, powders or coral calcium in tea
bags) can be argued to be somewhat indistinct. As we start to examine the specific chemical composition of coral calcium, its contents
of many elements in parts per million (very small amounts) will
become apparent.

ORIGINS OF THE SUGGESTIONS OF THE IMPOR-
TANCE OF BACTERIA IN CORAL CALCIUM

        Before we delve further into the hypotheses of how coral cal-
cium could exert a health benefit, certain fantasies must be further
dispelled. As previously discussed, some professed experts on coral
calcium claim that microorganisms (said to be present in coral calcium) play a role in the beneficial effect of coral calcium on health.
Reflect upon the descriptions of the processing of coral, which is
designed to render coral as sterile as possible. One may see imme-
diately the absurdity of this suggestion concerning the actions of
"microbes" in coral supplements. It has been stated that microorganisms in coral may help gastrointestinal function and "hearsay"
suggests that this theory was proposed by Scandinavian Scientists.
I can find no evidence to support this preposterous suggestion.
However, Dr. E. Enby MD, a Scandinavian physician, has proposed that much chronic disease may be related to undiscovered
infections in the body and he has linked this hypothesis to the presence of chronic acidity in the body. I believe that the confusion concerning the role of microorganisms linked to coral calcium may be
an ignorant interpretation of Dr. Enbys' assertions and work. I
stress that Dr. Enby has opinions (alternative thoughts) that may
not be shared by all practicing physicians.

BODY ACIDITY AND ALKALINITY

The whole issue of body acidity and alkalinity has become an issue of great debate in alternative and conventional medicine. Many practitioners of alternative medicine believe that modern lifestyle is pushing many people to a body status of acidity (low pH). It has been proposed that mineral intake, especially intake of "alkaline" metals (e.g. calcium), may assist in neutralizing the body acidity in a beneficial manner. Further, it has even been suggested that mineral intake may cause the body to become more alkaline. These hypotheses are very interesting, but they may be only "half-truths" (if one could accept a qualified truth!).

The body has very complex mechanisms that control acidity and alkalinity (pH balance in the body). Certainly this balance has much to do with many factors, other than mineral intake in the diet. With some naivety, people have recommended the monitoring of the pH (acidity or alkalinity) of certain body fluids (saliva and urine); and they have proposed that not only can body pH be influenced by mineral intake, one can give desirable amounts of minerals by gauging their effect on the pH of body fluids. I believe that this notion is "far-fetched". It must be recognized that body fluids have changes in pH (a measure of the presence of hydrogen ions, or acid) on a regular basis. For example, urine becomes alkaline after a meal. This is known in basic physiology as the "alkaline tide". Therefore, selling strips of paper (litmus paper) or gadgets to measure pH of body fluids as a way of monitoring the intake of minerals supplements has to be questioned. I am not suggesting that some minerals may not have a modest and positive influence on body pH, but I am suggesting that the influence is small in comparison to the many other systems in the body which act as the primary buffers of acid. I believe that selling products on the basis of balancing pH by using gadgets to measure body pH, such as litmus paper, strips, is quite misleading.

In summary, the main theories of how coral calcium works can be summarized as; a general natural holistic mineral supplement, or a homeopathic agent or cell salt therapy or as a regulator of body pH. I would add to these proposals the fact there may be other actions of coral calcium that remains undiscovered. Of the

proposed mechanisms of action for coral calcium and health, I favor
the explanation of the value of coral calcium as a natural mineral
supplement. As a mineral supplement, I believe that it provides a
wide range of available micronutrients (metals and minerals) that
support many body structures and functions. This explanation
makes most sense as people increasingly report that they "just feel
better" when they take coral calcium. This nonspecific report of
improvement and well-being could be explained by the overall value
of minerals for health, especially in individuals who may be depleted
of several micronutrient elements. The repaid swing of pH demonstrated by adding coral calcium enclosed in a tea bag to water may
often be related to the addition of "baking soda" (sodium bicarbonate) to the coral – a slick, sales trick!

ANALYZING CORAL CALCIUM

The most authoritative accounts of the analysis of fossilized,
stony coral minerals are to be found in the book by Dr. Bruce
Halstead, M.D. entitled "Fossil Stony Coral Minerals and Their
Nutritional Application" (a World Life Research Institute
Publication, 1999, available at www.wellnesspublishing.com). This
work antedates the publication of Mr. Barefoot's book (Barefoot
on Coral Calcium, www.wellnesspublishing.com). The analyses
of coral calcium performed by Dr. Halstead show most elemental
contents in parts per million, except for calcium and magnesium.
Dr. Halstead has summarized a comparison of major elements
found in the Earth's crust, seawater, human body and stony coral
fossils. He has reviewed the essential biological roles of the many
trace elements found in coral minerals (coral calcium).

THE MICRONUTRIENT CONTENT
OF CORAL CALCIUM

Whilst much has been made out of the importance of the
calcium and magnesium content of coral, much less discussion has
focused on the micronutrient mineral content of coral. Both marine
coral and land-based coral have a wide range of elements present
within them. In fact, land-based coral has been shown to have up

to 74 different elements on careful chemical analysis and marine coral may contain a similar range of elements.

Some researchers argue strongly that the micronutrient profile of land-based coral may be superior to marine coral. This is an unresolved debate. This observation has been proposed by some to counter the expressed opinion, that land-based coral is inferior in mineral content due to drying and leaching of metals and minerals. Examples of micronutrient analysis showing the content of various elements in coral is shown in table 3. These data are recent (September 2001) and they supersede other published material. Furthermore, I believe that the results to be particularly valuable because they were done by by independent laboratories, with no commercial interests in coral calcium.

BELOW-SEA COLLECTED CORAL (HIGHEST GRADE)

Calcium	20% or more
Magnesium	10% or more
Arsenic (as As)	2ppm or less
Heavy metal (as Ph)	0.5ppm or less
Size of Particle	44n m90%<
Pesticide residue	Undetectable (Endrin, Dildrin, Aldorin, BHC, DDT)

<Microorganisms>	
General bacteria count	3 x 10 (3)/g or less
Yeast	1 x 10 (2)/g or less
Mold	1 x 10 (2)/g or less
Colibacillus	Negative
Salmonella	Negative
Enteritis vibrio	Negative

ABOVE-SEA LEVEL COLLECTED CORAL CALCIUM (HIGHEST GRADE)

Calcium	35% or greater
Magnesium	6000 ppm or greater
Total minerals and elements	74 or greater
Lead	0.5 ppm or less
Mercury	0.1 ppm or less
Cadmium	0.3 ppm or less
Arsenic	0.5 ppm or less

Pesticide residue	Undetectable
Salmonella	Negative
Yeast	<10 cfu/g
Mold	<10 cfu/g
Total Coliform	<10 cfu/g
E. coli	<10 cfu/g

Table 3: The mineral profile and other relevant analyses of the content of the two highest grades of coral calcium used in dietary supplements. The data was supplied with the permission of Natures Benefit Inc. www.naturesbenefit.com. Both below-sea collected coral calcium and coral calcium collected above ground contain up to 70 or more micronutrient elements or minerals with natural marine variability. This micronutrient profile of types of coral calcium is displayed on the web page www.naturesbenefit.com. Many elements found in the earths crust are present in all forms of coral remnants and they are most frequently present in very small amounts, measured in parts per million. The below-sea collected coral carries a Japanese Food Research Laboratory certification, authorized by the Japanese Government. This product is used by Natures Benefit Inc. It is heat sterilized. The forms of above-sea collected coral remnants used by Natures Benefit Inc. are obtained from Okinawa and ground and processed in the USA. This form of coral is sterilized mainly by ozone treatment.

CONCERNS ABOUT SPECIFICATIONS ON CORAL

Whilst several sections of this short book may appear technical in its content, the information can be summarized in a simple manner.

First, the apparent advantage of some types of below-sea collected coral, appears to be a higher magnesium concentration. Second, the situation of low magnesium concentrations in some forms of coral calcium can be remedied and is often remedied by adding magnesium to coral. Third, in common with others, I cannot ascertain whether or not some of the processing companies in Japan add magnesium? (perhaps a moot point). Fourth, the reported health benefits from both types of high grade coral discussed in this book appear to be similar, with no credible evidence that below-sea collected coral calcium is superior or has an enhanced biological effect compared with land-based coral. Fifth, concerns must remain if manufacturers use below-sea collected coral with an excessive lead content. Sixth, the use of land-based coral may be, arguably, better for the environment.

MOVING TOWARDS THE IDEAL CORAL CALCIUM SUPPLEMENTS

How does this information transmit in to a recommendation for an ideal coral calcium supplement? The answer rests in considering the relative advantages or limitations of different types of coral calcium.

Therefore, it seems most appropriate for healthcare consumers to be offered land-based coral of high quality and below-sea coral of high quality to provide the consumer with choices and the relative advantages of both types of coral calcium (accepting that not all advantages and disadvantages may have been recognized to date, see www.naturesbenefit.com).

CORAL TEA BAGS

There has been a limited tradition in Western society of taking coral in "novel" our "unusual" formats. One popular way of taking coral is to drink coral water that has been exposed to a teabag containing coral powder with additives (sometimes "baking soda"). Mr. Barefoot has been very critical of this use of coral, although he once supported this form of coral "supplement". At first sight, criticism the use of coral water compared with encapsulated coral calcium seems plausible, because only a small percentage of coral minerals from the teabag dissolves in the water (less than 2 % over a matter of hours). It is obvious that swallowing coral calcium in whole capsules or powders as food additives provides greater amounts of mineral nutrients for the body. However, the advantages of coral teabags must not be dismissed lightly.

Dr. Bruce Halstead, M.D. has described the potential link between the presence of coral enriched water in Okinawa and the longevity of the local population. It would appear that the water supply in several areas of Okinawa is exposed to coral sand or fossilized remnants as a natural filtering mechanism. Casting our mind back to the homeopathic theory of the action of coral calcium, it could be hypothesized that coral water from coral enclosed teabags is a homeopathic medicine. My thoughts are speculations, but one could even imagine that Okinawa and its water supply is a massive homeopathic (or biochemic) healing environment, where other factors may operate to promote health and long life.

Many reported testimonials of the health benefits of using water exposed to coral calcium containing teabags have been displayed on the Internet. It is not clear, whether or not testimonials of the benefit of coral calcium in solid dosage forms (pills and powders) are confused with testimonials of health benefits from people using water treated with tea bag enclosed coral. I think that coral water is perceived by many people to be a convenient way of using coral calcium and coral material itself will assist in the removal of chlorine from water and tend to make the water alkaline.

DISSOLVING CORAL? WHAT NEXT?

Innovative manufacturers in Japan have now developed what they describe as a "dissolving-type" of coral calcium. This type of "dissolving coral" is sold in aluminum packages that are referred to as "coral calcium sticks." Apparently, this form of coral calcium has become popular in some European countries. I am puzzled by this product and even more puzzled by consumers, purveyors and self-proclaimed experts who think that coral calcium should dissolve completely in water.

Many minerals in coral calcium, e.g. calcium and magnesium, are in the "carbonate form". Carbonated minerals are relatively insoluble. In more simple terms, one can understand that if stony coral was able to dissolve completely in water, then there would be no coral reefs in the ocean! Recently, special encapsulation processes have been used to make liquid forms of coral calcium. I can see no advantage to this "novel" form of coral calcium which has little history of use and no credible precedent of health benefits.

SOME KEY BIOLOGICAL ACTIONS OF CORAL COMPONENTS

Dr. Bruce Halstead, M.D., a world renowned marine biologist and physician, has expressed the opinion that certain elements in coral minerals, such as deuterium or germanium may have novel health benefits. Dr. Halstead describes the presence of an approximate level of deuterium of 150 parts per million in stony fossilized corals. Elegant research by Dr. Halstead and others has shown that the chemical and biological actions of deuterium with organic molecules may be quite unique. Deuterium may bond with certain enzymes in a manner that is more stable than water bonds. There is an indication that these deuterium bonds may result in the enhancement of enzymatic reactions in the body (part of the chemistry of life) and this process may even enhance activity of many drugs. These theories are intriguing and I highly recommend that interested readers refer to Dr. Halstead's book (Fossil Stony Coral Minerals and their Nutritional Application, 1999, available at www.wellnesspublishing.com).

Dr. Halstead's book is an authoritative account of the biology of coral and he provides an interesting series of references that are relevant to an understanding of the actions of coral calcium. Such references are not found in other books on the subject of coral calcium. Dr. Halstead was a pioneer of research into chelation therapy and he believes that many minerals in coral calcium are naturally chelated. Chelated minerals afford advantages by the assimilation of minerals for the body. The word chelate comes from a Greek word that refers to the "claw" of a crab or lobster. In technical terms, it is the incorporation of a metal ion into a heterocyclic (chemical) ring structure. This kind of chemical binding process is described as a "bioinorganic" process. In simple terms, it may make elements more available for use by the body.

To avoid technicalities, one can perceive the chelation process in nature to be one of the important processes by which living organisms use metals. In brief, when minerals are chelated they are more effectively absorbed and utilized by living organisms. Thus, the presence of metals in coral in a chelated format may be another key to the understanding of the benefits of coral calcium as a mineral supplement.

A CLASH OF OPINION ON CORAL CALCIUM

Two differing opinions on the ideal form of coral minerals to use as a food or dietary supplement have emerged. On the one hand, Dr. Bruce W. Halstead MD (an icon in the field of marine biology and the treatment applications of marine nutraceuticals) believes that only coral collected above sea level should be used for human consumption. Dr. Halstead has made compelling arguments that fossilized stony minerals that reached land deposits many thousands of years ago contain bioactive chelated minerals which do not associate themselves with environmental pollutants. These are the pollutants that have emerged as a consequence of industrial revolutions in modern times. Furthermore, Dr. Halstead believes that stony coral minerals exert health benefits as a consequence of their global and specific micronutrient profile, not just as a consequence of the calcium content (or magnesium content) of coral remnants.

On the other hand, Robert Barefoot insists that the health benefits of coral calcium are related to its calcium content. His newfound, beliefs in the use of below-sea-level-collected coral remnants, which may have a 2:1 balance of calcium to magnesium as a "natural" consequence, are widely touted. The origin of the words "coral calcium" is unclear. I reiterate that the dietary supplement known as calcium appears to have much more to do with holistic micronutrient profiles in terms of its biological actions rather than just exerting a benefit through its content of calcium alone. Clearly, Mr. Barefoot and Dr. B. W. Halstead MD may not want to be mentioned in the same sentence, given their diametrically opposing view points. This clash of "Titans of Opinions" will be played out in the future.

The variability in opinions concerning the best type of coral calcium to use are clouded further by uninformed propaganda, emerging opinions to support different brands of coral calcium and major uncertainties about how coral calcium may work to provide a health benefit. The principal hypotheses proposed to explain the biomedical or biochemical actions of coral calcium include:

calcium content (a rejected concept by many)
balanced calcium and magnesium content (unlikely)
holistic mineral and elemental composition
    providing micronutrients (likely)
specific micronutrient metals (likely)
specific micronutrient elements e.g. deuterium (plausible)
alterations of body pH with a shift towards alkalinity
    (naïve component)
provision of a healthy balanced mineral intake (likely)
homeopathic activity (plausible)
Cell Salt Theory proposed initially by
    Dr. W. H. Schuessler (plausible)

I emphasize that the mechanism of action of coral calcium as a dietary supplement remains in question. The possibility that coral calcium exerts a benefit by a homeopathic mechanism or the biochemical expansion of homeopathic theory by Dr. W. H. Schuessler are my personal suggestions and represent hypotheses that I believe to be worthy of closer debate and examination.

CORAL CALCIUM AND HOMEOPATHY

Marine products (fish, coral etc.) have a long history of use in homeopathic medicines. However, their origin of these homeopathic medical ingredients are difficult to trace in history. Salts or minerals are a frequent inclusions in a large proportion of the many thousands of homeopathic formulae that are used to treat a wide variety of illnesses (see Boericke's Materia Medica). Homeopathic medicine was founded in the 18th Century by the celebrated physician Samuel Hahnemann. It was Dr. Hahnemann who reported great health significance and benefits, related to the use of mineral substances in minute amounts in homeopathic remedies. Several physicians have extended Dr. Hahnemann's original concepts of homeopathy and it was Dr. W. H. Schuessler (a renowned German physician) who extended standard homeopathic concepts to a system which he called "biochemistry" (biochemic) with an emphasis on this term representing "the chemistry of life".

Dr. W. H. Schuessler lived between the years 1821 and

1896. In 1880 Dr. Schuessler published his work with a translated title "Twelve Tissue Remedies". Dr. Schuesslers' treatment methods were not strictly examples of homeopathic treatments. He used twelve cell salts in his treatments, which have been variably described as biochemic salts, tissues remedies, colloids or simply "cell salts". These cell salts were considered by Dr. Schuessler to be essential for normal body function and he believed in a concept of restoration of vitality and balance to the body. These are not homeopathic concepts. Such concepts involve typically the principal of "like healing like" (similia similibus curantur). Dr. Schuessler believed that he was supplying the exact constituents that cells were lacking for normal biochemical functions.

Dr. Schuessler went further in his hypotheses. He was interested in astrology and linked each of the twelve cell salts with an astrological marker. In brief, the twelve cell salts are:

Silicea (Sagitarius)   Kali sulphuricum (Virgo)

Ferrum phosphoricum (Pisces)   Calcarea sulphuricum (Scorpio)

Natrum phosphorium (Libra)   Natrum muriaticum (Aquarius)

Kali phosphoricum (Aries)   Kali muriaticum (Gemini)

Natrum sulphuricum (Taurus)   Calcarea fluoricum (Cancer)

Calcarea phosphoricum   Magnesia phosphoricum (Leo).
(Capricorn)

Whilst Dr. Schuessler's twelve cell salts may be variably present in material like coral, there are major differences in elemental profiles between Schuesslers salts and coral calcium. However, Dr. Schuessler "potentized" his salts (a homeopathic technique). I find Dr. Schuessler's hypotheses consistent with how coral calcium could work, but not all homeopathic or other physicians believe in this "biochemic system" of treatment as proposed by Dr. Schuessler.

Other noted physicians have subscribed to Schuessler's hypotheses. One proponent was Dr. James H. Stephenson MD who died in 1985. Dr. Stephenson MD was a graduate of Cornell University. He became very interested in astrology and Schuessler's cell salts. Dr. Stephenson was mentored by the famous homeopathic expert, Elisabeth Wright Hubbard. Ms Hubbard had used Schuesslers' salts to cure Dr. Stephenson of chronic pain that he had developed whilst he was prisoner of war. In addition, the Australian homeopath Dr. M. Blackmore extended and popularized Schuessler's work in his book entitled "Celloids: A Textbook for Physicians" (1958). Dr. Blackmore claimed that he had "refined" Schuesslers' cell salt remedies by adding more substantial amounts and ranges of salts (except sodium chloride) to his remedies.

The most interesting account of the application of Schuesslers' remedies is to be found in the book entitled "Nature's 12 Magic Healers: The Amazing Secrets of Cell Salts" by Lionel Rolfe and Nigey Lennon (Parker Publishing Company Inc., West Nyack, New York, 1978). In this book, two eminent homeopathic physicians, Dr. J. H. Renner MD and Dr. William E. S. Jackson MD comment on the value of Schuesslers' cell salts. Dr. Kenner writes in a foreword *"Tissue salts are not a new, untried discovery. As a medical doctor with over fifty years of experience, I have used these tissue salts with results equal to those documented earlier. In these past two hundred years, results have been just fabulous"*.

Dr. Schuessler's reasoning may raise the eyebrows of the modern-day allopathic (conventional) physician, but Dr. Schuessler's system of cell salt therapies is widely practiced in modified formats in many countries, especially Germany. Dr. Schuessler reasoned that when a human cell is reduced to ashes, presumably by heat, there are only twelve minerals left. These twelve minerals were termed "cell salts", but there are more than twelve cell salts present. The reason for Dr. Schuessler's underestimate of the number of cell salts may have been related to limitations in his own laboratory analyses. Intuitively, Dr. Schuessler and his followers stated that a lack of basic cell salts will prevent nutrients entering cells to provide nourishment, with the result that normal body structure and function is not maintained and disease occurs. In general terms, Dr. Schuessler was proposing that lack of key cell salts in human diets created major imbalances in the body and interrupted what Dr. Claude Bernard (the famous French physiologist vicious and vivisectionist) had called "The Harmony of Life".

CALCIUM INTAKE: MULTIPLE BENEFITS

There are several recognized health benefits of calcium supplementation, other than the obvious effects of maintaining healthy bones. Calcium has been demonstrated to have a mild anti-hypertensive (blood-pressure lowering) effect. In one double-blind crossover study, people with moderate hypertension who received 1 gram per day of calcium for eight weeks had reductions in blood pressure during calcium administration. Reductions in blood lipids including cholesterol and triglycerides have been observed in long-term studies, thereby giving calcium a potential role in the promotion of cardiovascular wellness. Adequate calcium intake is known to play a valuable role in the prevention of cancer, especially colon cancer. It appears that calcium in the diet can prevent the recurrence of colon polyps. Polyps are pre-cancerous growths in the large bowel. Calcium deficiency may be associated with hundreds of diseases.

HEALTHY BONES: CLEAR BENEFITS FOR CALCIUM AND OTHER MINERALS

The beneficial effects of calcium supplementation on bone intensity and bone loss in premenopausal and postmenopausal, "middle-aged women" is well recognized. Several studies in Western society have shown that women have a loss of bone density when they have a daily calcium consumption of less than 400 mg/day. Loss of bone density tends to be much less in women who have a calcium intake of approximately 750mg/day or more. Even though some scientific studies have failed to show a major beneficial effect of calcium supplementation in preventing or reversing osteoporosis, an overwhelming body of opinion is in favor of calcium supplementation as a preventive measure for osteoporosis.

AMOUNTS AND TYPES OF DIETARY CALCIUM

Accepting the importance of dietary calcium supplementation, the amount and chemical type of calcium and the source and format of calcium in the diet are believed to be important variables in the promotion of general and bone health. Calcium carbonate is the most frequently used salt of calcium in dietary supplement preparations and calcium is present as carbonate in coral calcium. However, experts believe that the natural origin of calcium in coral calcium (or other natural sources of calcium e.g. egg-shell calcium) presents advantages (e.g. Dr. Halsteads' hypotheses about chelation). Calcium supplements should be taken with food to provide optimal absorption into the body. Contrary to popular belief, relatively insoluble salts of calcium, such as calcium carbonate, can be absorbed in the relative absence of gastric acid; even though absorption is less efficient.

I believe that an optimal amount of calcium to be taken in the diet of most people is 800 – 1000 mg/day for average adults and about 1-2g/day for young or "mature" and elderly adults. Several studies have indicated that calcium intake in many diets may often be below the RDA, especially in the elderly. Only about one quarter of all children of school age receive an optimum amount of calcium in their diet. The ideal way to supplement calcium in the diet is to eat calcium-rich foods but the range of such foods is limited and dietary supplements represent a convenient and consistent source of calcium. There are several adverse effects of taking too much calcium in the diet, especially if an individual is otherwise not healthy and particularly if renal (kidney) failure is present. However, there is some emerging evidence that taking calcium from natural sources (e.g. coral calcium and egg shell calcium) may lead to less adverse effects from high blood calcium (hypercalcemia, see www.antiporosis.com).

REVISITING CALCIUM SUPPLEMENTS

An increased intake of calcium from calcium-rich foods is required by many people, including these taking coral calcium at current recommended daily intakes of 1.5 g/day (1500 mg). Increasing calcium intake is often a difficult feat for many people on an average American diet. A list of calcium-rich foods is shown in table 4.

FOOD	CALCIUM AMOUNT	CONTENT (mg)
Sardines with bones	? cup	500
Mackerel with bones	? cup	300
Milk	1 cup	288
Fortified rice milk	1 cup	280
Broccoli	1 cup	178
Mustard greens, cooked	1 cup	180
Canned red salmon	? cup	275
Fortified soy milk	1 cup	280
Cooked brown rice	1 cup	20
Cooked oats	1 cup	40
Lentils	1 cup	50
Black beans	1 cup	60
Walnuts	? cup	70
Hazelnuts	? cup	115
Soybeans	1 cup	130
Tofu	1 cup	150
Lima beans	1 cup	60
Alfalfa sprouts	1 cup	25
Romaine lettuce	1 cup	40
Almonds	? cup	175

Table 4: A list of calcium containing foods with their approximate calcium content.

The emphasis placed on milk and dairy products as a good source of calcium requires cautious interpretation. Whole milk and dairy products contain unwanted calories, a high content of saturated fat and cholesterol. Furthermore, milk protein allergies are a significant issue. It is notable that several scientists have highlighted the potential of food allergies (e.g. milk protein allergy) as a potential cause of osteoporosis, and other chronic diseases, but this is arguable.

EXAMINING OTHER DIETARY SUPPLEMENT SOURCES OF CALCUM

There has been much debate about the ideal form of calcium supplement to take and table 5 addresses some the advantages and limitations of several forms of calcium that are used as dietary supplements.

Type of Calcium	Concentration Calcium	Advantages	Disadvantages
Microcrystalline Hydroxyapatite	25%	Well absorbed complete bone food, absorbed by those with poor digestion	Costly source for elemental calcium, may contain toxic heavy metals
Citrate	24%	Well absorbed, may reduce the risk of kidney stones	A lot needs to be used in a supplement because of low calcium concentration
Di-Calcium Phosphate Calcium Concentration	28%	Advantage of calcium to phosphorus ratio. inexpensive form of elemental calcium	Not well absorbed in patients with high dietary phosphorus intakes, may further distort normal calcium to phosphorus levels
Lactate	15%	Well absorbed. Expensive source of elemental calcium	May contain allergens e.g. yeast and milk protein from fermentation processes.
Carbonate	40%	Least expensive form of calcium, highest content of elemental calcium	Variable absorption, may create gastric distress (switches on acid secretion in stomach and causes constipation).

Bone Meal	39%	Complete bone food rich source of elemental calcium	May contain toxic levels of lead, arsenic, and cadmium. Organic constituents are destroyed in processing
Coral Calcium	24-42%	More than calcium, up to 70 "micronutrient" minerals. best taken in ratio of 2:1 calcium to magnesium. No tendency to cause hyper-calcemia	Cost, but it is more than just a calcium supplement.
Egg Shell Calcium (Miracal™)	35-40%	A very attractive form of Calcium supplement, well absorbed and inexpensive. reduced tendency to cause hypercalcemia	None

Table 5: Types of calcium supplements: their advantages and disadvantages.

Whilst much debate has occurred about the best form of calcium to take as a supplement, many advantages have been proposed for forms of calcium from natural sources. These forms of calcium produced by living organisms have been particularly favored. Exciting new options involve the use of calcium form coral (coral calcium) and the use of calcium from egg shells (www.miracal.com).

SCIENTIFIC STUDIES OF CORAL CALCIUM

Studies performed at the University of Rukuyuku and the University of Okinawa have shown that calcium absorption from coral calcium into the body of experimental animals was better than absorption of calcium from milk-associated-calcium and cow-bone derived calcium (hydroxyapatite), see table 6. These feeding experiments in animals were carefully controlled and the organs and blood of the animals were analyzed for calcium and magnesium contents. An incidental finding in these studies was a favorable change in blood cholesterol. This type of coral calcium is used in the products Barefoot Coral Calcium Plus™, Marine Coral Minerals™ in 1.5 gram per day amounts. Assertions that calcium is 100% absorbed from coral calcium are frankly untrue.

	Control Group	Coral Minerals	Milk	Cow Bone
Calcium (Ca)				
Intake (mg/3 days)	319.3 +/- 13.9	360.2 +/- 6.3	313.2 +/- 6.4	318.9 +/- 15.4
Absorption (mg/3 days)	177.8 +/- 7.7	251.6 +/- 15.1	195.3 +/- 7.0	213.8 +/- 12.8
Percent (%) Absorption	55.9 +/- 2.1	69.6 +/- 3.1	62.4 +/- 1.8	66.9 +/- 1.4
Magnesium (Mg)				
Intake (mg/3 days)	131.0 +/- 5.7	161.8 +/- 2.8	131.2 +/- 2.7	161.7 +/- 7.8
Absorption (mg/3 days)	70.1 +/- 3.4	117.9 +/- 5.0	66.6 +/- 4.3	109.6 +/- 6.4
Percent (%) Absorption	53.6 +/- 1.6	72.8 +/- 2.3	50.8 +/- 3.2	69.7 +/- 1.8
Phosphorus (P)				
Intake (mg/3 days)	278.3 +/- 12.1	316.8 +/- 5.5	279.3 +/- 7.3	273.2 +/- 13.2
Absorption (mg/3 days)	107.6 +/- 8.2	267.7 +/- 6.9	192.1 +/- 3.4	177.7 +/- 9.5
Percent (%) Absorption	71.1 +/- 1.5	84.5 +/- 1.1	68.8 +/- 1.1	65.2 +/- 2.9

Table 6: The absorption of calcium from coral calcium in these experiments was superior to the absorption of calcium from several other forms of calcium supplements. Calcium, Magnesium and Phosphorus Absorption Rates are shown.

Two Japanese researchers (S. Kawamura and T. Taniuchi) have written an illuminating account of the use of calcium supplements, including coral calcium in their book "Warning! Calcium deficiency" (Shundaiyoyosha Publishing Co., Tokyo, Japan, 1999). These researchers reported a 30 year study with 20,000 case histories concerning more than forty different, over-the-counter, calcium supplements. They found that people taking large amounts of ionized calcium often experienced adverse symptoms due to high blood calcium levels (hypercalcemia). They noted that rapid swings in blood calcium could occur with occasional abrupt lowering of blood calcium in individuals taking calcium supplements (hypocalcemia). These Japanese scientists found that individuals who took coral calcium or other marine calcium products did not tend to suffer from states of high or low blood calcium. The lack of gyration of blood calcium when taking coral calcium is a real advantage, according to the aforementioned Japanese scientists.

Dr. Kunihiko Ishitani and colleagues report the superior absorption of calcium from the intake of coral calcium added to food in 1999 in J. Nutr. Sci. Vitaminol., 45, 509-517. In this small but well controlled study, these Japanese researchers used coral calcium powder containing crackers and compared them with plain calcium carbonate containing crackers, in terms of the ability of a small number of subjects (6 men and 6 women) to absorb calcium from the dietary intake of these crackers. In brief, the amount of intestinal absorption of calcium from crackers containing coral calcium (containing calcium to magnesium in a ratio of 2:1) was greater than the absorption of calcium from crackers containing only calcium carbonate. There was wide variability in the amount of calcium absorbed in these subjects used in the studies, regardless of whether or not coral calcium containing crackers or calcium carbonate containing crackers were eaten. The authors of this study referred to a study by Dr. K. Suzuki and colleagues, presented in 1997 and referred to previously as showing enhanced absorption of calcium in rats from coral calcium in comparison with a number of other forms of calcium (Suzuki K et al, Calcium utilization from natural coral calcium – A coral preparation with a calcium-magnesium content ratio of 2:1. Abstracts of Papers Presented at the 44th Jpn. Soc. Nutr. Betterment, p. 145, Fukuoka). The authors of these two studies claim that the Ryukyu Islands of Okinawa yield coral with approximately 20% and 10% calcium and magnesium content, respectively, but whether or not this coral is blended is not entirely clear.

CORAL CALCIUM AND OSTEOPOROSIS

Scientific studies performed at the Futaba Nutrition School of the Kagawa Nutrition University in Japan show the benefit of coral calcium in improvements in bone mineral density given in a balanced composition of 600 mg of calcium with 300 mg of magnesium (calcium:magnesium, 2:1 ratio). This research study was presented at the 52nd Japanese Society of Nutrition and Food

Science (April, 1998). In this well-conducted study, there were six experimental groups of subjects. These groups were:

A group receiving coral calcium and low-fat milk as calcium reinforcement in the diet.

A group taking the same calcium reinforcement in the diet with exercise in first period of study in the form of strength training and in the third period walking.

A group taking the same calcium reinforcement with exercise in the first period as walking and in the third period strength as training.

A group engaged in exercise only as in 2 above.

A group engaged in exercise only as in 3 above.

A control group.

These carefully performed studies show that all experimental groups, except the control group showed increases in bone mineral density. The greatest change in bone mineral density was shown in group 2 who took calcium reinforcement with milk and coral calcium, together with exercise consisting of initial strength training followed later in the study by walking. This study is highly relevant to the fundamental components of products that use coral calcium to build bone density (see the Antiporosis Plan by S. Holt, www.wellnesspublishing.com). The product Antiporosis™ uses a unique form of calcium supplementation with a combination of coral calcium and egg shell calcium ("Miracal™). The Antiporosis Plan recommends nutrition and lifestyle change, especially exercise for the management of osteoporosis (see www.naturesbenefit.com and www.antiporosis.com).

RETURNING TO THE IMPORTANCE
OF VITAMIN D

The biochemistry of vitamin D is very complex. Calcium works together with vitamin D (especially vitamin D3) and neither nutrient can be effective without each other. A substantial proportion of calcium absorption into the body is under the control of vitamin D3. This vitamin exerts major influences on the handling of calcium (metabolism) by the body. Whilst some controversy has existed concerning the bone building actions of calcium and vitamin D in osteoporosis, many scientific studies point to the benefits of this vital combination of nutrients (especially in senile or elderly-type osteoporosis).

When the levels of vitamin D fall in the body, the blood levels of calcium will tend to fall and calcium cannot be laid down in bone. A deficiency of vitamin D causes a specific bone disease called osteomalcia, where there is insufficient calcium in bones making them rubbery and weak. This disorder is called "rickets" (osteomalacia) and it is a different disease than osteoporosis. Rickets can cause many skeletal deformities (e.g. bumps on bones, bow-legs). The disease of Rickets has been largely eradicated by fortification of foods with vitamin D.

Vitamin D is synthesized in the body as a consequence of exposure to sunshine (an ultimate "nutrient"). A lack of exposure to sunshine made the disease of rickets a particular problem in several groups of people (e.g. underground workers, coal miners, the elderly who are housebound etc.). Vitamin D deficiency plays a major role in senile osteoporosis (osteoporosis of the elderly) which is quite often responsive to vitamin D administration and adequate, but safe, exposure to sunlight.

Deficiencies of vitamin D will cause bone to lose calcium because as blood levels of calcium fall then calcium is taken from the "calcium bank" in bones. The recommended daily intake of vitamin D is 200 international units, but many studies have shown advantages of extra vitamin D in certain groups of individuals. However, the taking off excessive amounts of vitamin D should be carefully monitored because vitamin D is toxic when taken in excess. Vitamin D is a major component of the "Antiporosis Plan" to combat osteoporosis; and when taken in modest doses in combination with calcium (www.antiporosis.com) and other bone building nutrients it is highly beneficial for individuals wishing to prevent or treat osteoporosis.

THE SUNLIGHT SAGA

Vitamin D is active in its D3 form which is synthesized in the skin as a consequence of sunlight. On the one hand, sunlight exposure is necessary and healthy for vitamin D synthesis, but on the other hand, modern science has clearly defined the health risks of overexposure to the sun. Recommendations, by some alternative healthcare givers, that hours of unprotected sun exposure is health-giving must be considered "patent nonsense".

Medical science has recorded that factors that limit exposure to sunlight are useful in the prevention of premature skin aging and cancer. However, very limited sun exposure can diminish the body status of vitamin D and, on occasion, secondarily exert a negative effect on bone health. Healthy sun exposure should be controlled exposure and this casual type of exposure will meet most of the body's vitamin D requirement, in most climates, in most people. It appears that it is only the elderly in Western communities that may be at risk of vitamin D deficiency due to a lack of sunlight exposure.

MORE ON MAGNESIUM

The role of magnesium in the support of bone structure and function has been grossly underestimated. More than one half of all of the body's magnesium is found in bone tissue where it exerts multiple effects on body chemistry that controls bone health. A deficiency of magnesium may result in a tissue resistance to the actions of vitamin D3 and parathyroid hormone; and it may cause an interference with the release of parathyroid hormone. Despite the known importance of magnesium for bone health, there have been relatively few studies on the ability of magnesium supplements to increase bone density in people with osteoporosis, or other chronic diseases. Magnesium has many beneficial effects on cardiovascular function and it is an important enzyme co-factor. In one important study in people with malabsorption due to celiac disease (a sensitivity to gluten from wheat, a food allergy), magnesium supplements were shown to improve blood levels of parathyroid hormone and cause increases in bone density. The higher magnesium content of the form of coral or the addition of magnesium salts to coral may have some advantages.

THE HEALTH BENEFITS OF CORAL CALCIUM

There are now thousands of testimonials on the health benefits of coral calcium, but no controlled scientific studies have emerged. Robert Barefoot believes that coral calcium has panacea benefits for health. In addition, Dr. Bruce Halstead has emphasized the health benefits of fossilized coral minerals. Whilst I have attempted to pinpoint the mechanism(s) of the health benefits of Okinawan, coral calcium material, no single consensus opinion exists. In summary, I favor the notion that coral calcium is a valuable holistic mineral supplement. It has apparent potent and versatile health benefits that require much more research and systematized documentation. The putative benefits of coral calcium are displayed on the world wide web (internet) by many people, as are the comments of the skeptics.

THE OKINAWA PROGRAM

The excellent book entitled "The Okinawa Program" (2000), written by BJ Willcox MD, D Craig Willcox PhD and Makoto Suzuki MD describes how Okinawan people may achieve their longevity. The celebrated practitioner of alternative medicine, Dr. Andrew Weil MD writes his own observations on how Okinawans may enjoy healthy and long life in the foreword to "The Okinawa Program". Both the authors of this book and Dr. Weil describe the notable differences between the people of Okinawa and the mainland Japanese and Westerners. This book focuses upon many aspects of lifestyle that are known to be associated with health and long life. These factors include a good level of physical activity, the eating of fish and soy foods with abundant fruits and vegetables. The social interactions in Okinawa and the sense of community spirit gives Okinawan people an apparently greater "self-responsibility" for their health, according to Dr. Weil.

While the authors stress the importance of vitamin and minerals intake for health. This book on the longevity of Okinawan people is not focused on the use of coral calcium. However, the research of the Okinawa Program has shown that higher levels of lifelong calcium intake may have occurred in the elite elderly (centenarians). Dr. Bradley J. Willcox MD and his colleagues indicate that men and women in Okinawa that have reached centenarian status may obtain about 625 mg and 400 mg of calcium from food, on a respective basis. These scientists do stress that Okinawan people obtain a significant amount of calcium from their drinking water due to the presence of coral deposits on the islands. The authors of "The Okinawa Program" cite the book entitled "A Professional Handbook of Complementary and Alternative Medicine", published by Springhouse Corporation, PA, 1999, as a reference that hip fracture rates are low in Okinawa largely as a consequence of the calcium from coral deposits that is present in drinking water in Okinawa. Readers are requested to reflect on opinions that coral calcium can exert most of its benefits in terms of being "the calcium factor". Clearly, the science of the "Okinawan Program" does not link longevity directly to coral calcium intake.

FACTOIDS

Many consumers of coral calcium are confused by inaccurate statements about the composition and potential biological actions of coral calcium (marine coral minerals or fossilized stony coral minerals). The following facts and conclusions from available information may help dispel some of the "marketing mumbo-jumbo" on coral calcium:

1) Testimonials of the benefits of coral calcium are not "proof" of a consistent, beneficial health effect. However, the volume of testimonials of benefits cannot be ignored and should be further explored. The continuing use of coral calcium by many people as a consequence of their perceived benefit is an important issue.
2) Calcium contained in coral calcium is not 100% absorbed, nor is it completely ionized in the human gastrointestinal tract in most people.
3) Coral calcium supplements do not contain "microbes". They are treated in a manner that eliminates bacteria, fungi molds and other living material. Marine "microbes" are not "probiotic" agents with beneficial effects on the human gastrointestinal tract.

4) Whilst the magnesium content of coral collected below-sea level may be higher than coral collected above-sea level, a consistent balance of calcium to magnesium of 2:1 does not occur in nature in the coral sand precursor of the dietary supplement coral calcium. Below-sea collected coral is probably "blended" to bring up the magnesium content to 12%, approximately.

5) There is no clear evidence, whatsoever, to state that below-sea collected coral sand results in a more effective coral calcium supplement. Some evidence suggests that above-sea level collected coral calcium is more suitable for use as a supplement, at least in terms of both safety and efficacy. These matters remain unresolved.

6) Statements that coral calcium cures or prevents cancer are not scientific facts. The media statements that individuals can "grow new brains" or cure degenerative neurological illness, such as Parkinson's Disease are absurd remarks.

7) Coral calcium probably works by mechanisms other than its content of calcium alone (see Dr. Bruce Halstead's work).

8) Mr. Robert Barefoot, the author of the book "Barefoot on Coral Calcium: An Elixir of Life", is neither a medical practitioner nor a doctor of biomedical scientist. He is a chemist who worked in the petroleum industry. Dr. Bruce Halstead MD is a highly experienced, marine biologist, medical doctor and expert in the health applications of marine products or materials. He has written one of the most valuable, extensive documents on marine toxicology that has been used by several governments. Dr. Halstead MD believes that only above sea-collected coral should be used for coral calcium supplements (see the book "Fossilized Stony Coral Minerals and their Nutritional Application by B. Halstead MD).

9) Several companies claim that Mr. Barefoot has donated his likeness (sometimes on an exclusive basis) to sell coral calcium supplements. Mr. Robert Barefoot has variably promoted and endorsed the use of coral calcium in all forms: above-ground collected, below-sea collected and tea bag enclosed coral to make coral water. Currently, he seems to favor below-sea collected coral. Several disputes have arisen over the use of Mr. Barefoot's likeness, especially in rela-

tionship to TV commercials.

10) The use of coral calcium should be guided by fact, not speculation. Much about the benefits, or lack thereof, of coral calcium remains unknown. The use of coral calcium should not be guided by a likeness, personality or endorsement.

11) At the time of writing, the only company that provides both forms of coral (above and below-sea collected coral sand) in four clearly labeled products is Natures Benefit Inc. and specifications of these products are published on the internet at www.naturesbenefit.com and www.coralcalciuminformation.com.

12) Books written on the subject of coral calcium are not to be confused as labels on products. They represent only authors' opinions (including this book!).

13) Testimonials in the use of coral calcium do not often define the type of coral calcium used e.g. by brand, by type, by delivery (above-sea or below-sea collected in capsules or enclosed in tea bags). Some coral calcium is cut with "fillers".

14) Much misleading information exists on the internet and in books written on the subject of coral calcium. Many internet sites promise cures of diseases with coral calcium and whilst these "cures" may have appeared in testimonials, there are no controlled clinical trials on specific disease treatments with coral calcium.

15) Coral calcium is a valuable, natural holistic mineral supplement, containing many potential micronutrients.

16) Whilst magnesium intake is important calcium and magnesium compete for absorption. This means that magnesium can interfere with calcium absorption and vice versa.

17) Recommendations for high doses of vitamin D are dangerous and with continued use serious toxicity may occur.

18) No evidence exists to support the use of cesium, nickel or silver as "nutritional" supplements. These are toxic elements at significant levels of intake or with chronic continued use. Cesium is not a proven cancer cure.

19) Uncontrolled, excessive exposure to sunlight is damaging to health.

20) Dr. Otto Warburg did not have coral calcium in mind when he described his Nobel Prize winning research Calcium intake is not a primary way of supplying oxygen the body.

21) Measurements of the pH of body fluids is not an accurate, reproducible or even useful way of gauging the intake of minerals. Measurements of the pH of saliva for guiding mineral supplement intake are probably valueless. Coral tea bags that show rapid shifts in the pH of water towards alkalinity may often contain "baking soda" (sodium bicarbonate) or calcinated coral sand (sodium bicarbonate). The actual contents of some tea bags containing coral are not always listed on labels.

22) Coral calcium does not "dissolve" in water.

23) The Food and Drug Administration provides a valuable public service and it does not condone treatment claims on supplements.

24) Companies that sell coral calcium with treatment claims must be avoided.

25) Many types of coral calcium are sold. These dietary supplements differ in their manufacture, additives etc. The term coral calcium is not an accurate description of coral minerals used as a dietary supplement. Coral minerals are a source of many minerals, often in small amounts.

26) Mr. Barefoot states "all coral is fantastic". This may not be the case.

27) Dr. B. Halstead MD believes that the micronutrient (elemental) trace components of coral calcium exert important biological effects. This may or may not be the case.

28) The only significant scientific observations on the use of coral calcium in potential disease management relate to osteoporosis.

29) Whilst the presence of coral calcium in the environment of Okinawa "may" contribute to longevity, many other factors operate.

30) Many people claim a benefit from taking coral calcium – a fact. More research is required to assess these reports of benefit.

THE CONSUMERS CHOICE OF CORAL CALCIUM

I have purposely avoided any lengthy discussion of testimonials on the health benefits of coral calcium. Some people argue that these testimonials are proof of benefit, whilst others demand controlled scientific studies as proof of health benefits. When it comes to choosing a coral calcium supplement there are several important issues to address.

First, the coral calcium supplement should be clearly labeled and ideally the source of coral calcium should be identified, but this has not occurred consistently. Second, the coral calcium supplement should be food grade and it should not contain toxic heavy metals or organic pollutants. Third, forms of coral calcium supplements for which there is a precedent of beneficial use should be used. Whilst these general principles apply without argument, there are at least twenty five brands of coral calcium available in the US market, differing in source, dosage processing and delivery (see www.wellnesspublishing.com and www.naturesbenefit.com).

In conclusion, the mechanism of action of coral calcium as a health giving supplement remains in doubt. High quality coral calcium fossils collected from below or above the sea level appear to have equivalent health benefits, but more studies are required. That said, the benefits reported by the thousands of people taking coral calcium supplements cannot be ignored. Consumers must be given a choice of high grade coral supplements, but more important, they must be given accurate information in order to make an "informed choice" (www.naturesbenefit.com, www.coralcalciuminformation.com). What is most impressive is the continuity of use of this important mineral supplement by many consumers. This continuity of use has occurred largely as a consequence of benefits among consumers of selected coral calcium dietary supplements. Coral calcium is here to stay as an underexplored, valuable dietary supplement that must not be misunderstood.

REFERENCES:

Asai K, *Miracle Cure. Organic germanium*, Japan Publications, Tokyo – cited by B. Halstead MD.

Barefoot R, Barefoot *On Coral Calcium: An Elixir of Life*, Wellness Publishing, www.wellnesspublishing.com, 2001.

Bianchi CF, *Cell Calcium*. Appleton – Century Crofts, London, 1968.

Boericke OE, *Boericke Pocket Manual of Homeopathic Material Medica with Repertory*, B. Jain Publishers Letd. New Delhi, 1992 (reprint edition).

Curtin ME, *Chemicals from the Sea*, Biotechnology, 3, 1, 34, 36-37, 1985.

Der Marderosian A, Liberti L, *Natural Product Miedicine*, George F. Stickley Co, PA, 1988.

Faulkner DJ, *Marine Natural Products*, Natural Product Reports, 3, 1, 1-33, 1986.

Faulkner D, Chesher R, *Living Corals*, CN Potter Inc., NY, 1979.

Halstead BW and CL Foster, *Drugs from the sea*, Chinese J. Mar. Drugs, 9(1):1-32, 1990.

Halstead BW and TC Rozema, *The Scientific Basis of EDTA Chelation Therapy*, TRC Publishing, Landrum, SC, 1997.

Halstead BW, *Fossil Stony Coral Minerals and Their Nutritional Application*, Health Digest Publishing Company, Cannon Beach, Oregon, 1999.

Halstead BW, *Poisonous and Venemous Marine Animals of the World*, The Darwin Press Inc., Princeton, NJ, 1988.

Halstead BW, *The Sceintific Basis of EDTA Chelation Therapy*, Golden Quill Press, Colton, CA, 1979.

Holliday L, Wood E, *Coral reefs*, Salamander Books, New York, 1989.

Holt S, Bader D, *Natures Benefit For Pets*, Wellness Publishing.

Holt S, Barilla JR, *The Power of Cartilage*, Kensington Publishers, NY, NY, 1998.

Holt S, Comac L, *Miracle Herbs*, Carol Publishing, NJ, 1997.

Holt S, *Natural Ways to Digestive Health*, M. Evans Inc., NY, NY, 2000.

Holt S, *The Natural Way to a Healthy Heart*, M. Evans Inc., NY, NY,1999.

Holt S, *The Soy Revolution*, Dell Publishing, Random House, NY, NY, 1999.

Kent JT, *Repertory of the Homeopathic Materia Medica with Word Index*, B. Jain Publishers Ltd, New Delhi, 1991.

Kobyashi J, *The Secret of Health and Longevity in Okinawa*, The Sokai, Okinawa, 1990 – cited by B. W. Halstead.

NIH, *Optimal Calcium Intake*, National Institutes of Health, 12, 4, 1-24, 1994.

Rolfe L, Lennon N, *Nature's 12 Magic Healers: The Amazing Secrets of Cell Salts*, Parker Publishing Company, Inc., West Nyack, NY, 1978.

Scheuer P, *Chemistry of Marine Natural Products*, Academic Press, NY, 1973.

Ullman D, *Discovering Homeopathy*, North Atlantic Books, Berkely, CA, 1991.

Willcox BJ, Willcox DC, Makoto Suzuki, *The Okinawa Program: How the world's longest-lived people achieve everlasting health – and how you can too*, Clarkson Potter/Publishers, NY, NY, 2000.

Web sites:

www.wellnesspublishing, books on coral calcium.
www.naturesbenefit.com, commercial sources of coral calcium.
www.coralcalciuminformation.com, up to date information.
www.antiporosis.com, commercial information on coral calcium for bone health
www.calciodecoral.net, commercial information in Spanish.
www.antiagingmethods.com, prevent premature death.
www.combatsyndromeX.com, the most important public health initiative.